T0259245

Production Animal Ophthalmology

Guest Editor

DAVID L. WILLIAMS, MA, VetMB, PhD, CertVOphthal, FRCVS

VETERINARY CLINICS OF NORTH AMERICA: FOOD ANIMAL PRACTICE

www.vetfood.theclinics.com

Consulting Editor
ROBERT A. SMITH, DVM, MS

November 2010 • Volume 26 • Number 3

SAUNDERS an imprint of ELSEVIER, Inc.

W.B. SAUNDERS COMPANY
A Division of Elsevier Inc.

1600 John F. Kennedy Boulevard • Suite 1800 • Philadelphia, PA 19103-2899

http://www.vetfood.theclinics.com

VETERINARY CLINICS OF NORTH AMERICA: FOOD ANIMAL PRACTICE Volume 26, Number 3
November 2010 ISSN 0749-0720, ISBN-13: 978-1-4377-2505-6

Editor: John Vassallo; j.vassallo@elsevier.com
Developmental Editor: Jessica Demetriou

Veterinary Clinics of North America: Food Animal Practice (ISSN 0749-0720) is published in March, July, and November by Elsevier Inc., 360 Park Avenue South, New York, NY 10010-1710. Subscription prices are $199.00 per year (domestic individuals), $278.00 per year (domestic institutions), $93.00 per year (domestic students/residents), $225.00 per year (Canadian individuals), $363.00 per year (Canadian institutions), $284.00 per year (international individuals), $363.00 per year (international institutions), and $142.00 per year (international and Canadian students/residents). To receive student/resident rate, orders must be accompanied by name of affiliated institution, date of term, and the signature of program/residency coordinator on institution letterhead. *Clinics* subscription prices. All prices are subject to change without notice. **POSTMASTER:** Send address changes to *Veterinary Clinics of North America*: *Food Animal Practice*, Elsevier Health Sciences Division, Subscription Customer Service, 3251 Riverport Lane, Maryland Heights, MO 63043. Customer Service (orders, claims, online, change of address): Elsevier Health Sciences Division, Subscription Customer Service, 3251 Riverport Lane, Maryland Heights, MO 63043. Tel: 1-800-654-2452 (U.S. and Canada); 314-447-8871 (ouside U.S. and Canada). Fax: 314-447-8029. E-mail: journalscustomerservice-usa@elsevier.com (for print support); journalsonlinesupport-usa@elsevier.com (for online support).

Reprints. For copies of 100 or more, of articles in this publication, please contact the Commercial Reprints Department, Elsevier Inc., 360 Park Avenue South, New York, NY 10010-1710. Tel.: 212-633-3812; Fax: 212-462-1935; E-mail: reprints@elsevier.com.

Veterinary Clinics of North America: Food Animal Practice is covered in *Current Contents/Agriculture, Biology and Environmental Sciences, MEDLINE/PubMed (Index Medicus), and Excerpta Medica.*

Printed and bound by CPI Group (UK) Ltd, Croydon, CR0 4YY
Transferred to Digital Print 2011

Contributors

CONSULTING EDITOR

ROBERT A. SMITH, DVM, MS
Diplomate, American Board of Veterinary Practitioners; Veterinary Research and Consulting Services, LLC, Greeley, Colorado

GUEST EDITOR

DAVID L. WILLIAMS, MA, VetMB, PhD, CertVOphthal, CertWEL, FRCVS
Associate Lecturer, Veterinary Ophthalmology and Animal Welfare, Department of Veterinary Medicine, University of Cambridge, Cambridge, United Kingdom

AUTHORS

DOMINIC ALEXANDER, BVMS, CBiol, MSB, MRCVS
Belmont Veterinary Centre; Cambridge Infectious Diseases Consortium (Clinical Research Outreach Programme), Department of Veterinary Medicine, University of Cambridge, Cambridge, United Kingdom

JOHN A. ELLIS, DVM, PhD
Diplomate, American College of Veterinary Pathologists; Diplomate, American College of Veterinary Microbiologists (Virology, Immunology); Professor, Department of Veterinary Microbiology, Western College of Veterinary Medicine, University of Saskatchewan, Saskatoon, Saskatchewan, Canada

HIDAYET METIN ERDOGAN, DVM, PhD
Professor of Internal Diseases, Division of Veterinary Clinical Science, Department of Internal Diseases, Faculty of Veterinary Medicine, University of Kafkas, Kars, Turkey

JULIET R. GIONFRIDDO, DVM, MS
Diplomate, American College of Veterinary Ophthalmologists; Associate Professor of Veterinary Ophthalmology, Department of Clinical Sciences, College of Veterinary Medicine and Biomedical Sciences, Veterinary Medical Center, Colorado State University, Fort Collins, Colorado

SHELDON MIDDLETON, MA, VetMB, MRCVS
Acorn House Veterinary Surgery, Linnet Way, Brickhill, Bedford, United Kingdom

CARYN E. PLUMMER, DVM
Diplomate, American College of Veterinary Ophthalmologists; Assistant Professor, Comparative Ophthalmology Service, Departments of Small and Large Animal Sciences, University of Florida, College of Veterinary Medicine, Gainesville, Florida

RACHEL SHAW-EDWARDS, BA, VetMB, MRCVS
Department of Veterinary Medicine, University of Cambridge, Cambridge, United Kingdom

WENDY M. TOWNSEND, DVM, MS
Diplomate, American College of Veterinary Ophthalmologists; Assistant Professor,
Comparative Ophthalmology, Department of Small Animal Clinical Sciences,
Michigan State University, East Lansing, Michigan

HIROKI TSUJITA, DVM
Chief Resident, Comparative Ophthalmology Service, Departments of Small and Large
Animal Sciences, University of Florida, College of Veterinary Medicine, Gainesville, Florida

DAVID L. WILLIAMS, MA, VetMB, PhD, CertVOphthal, CertWEL, FRCVS
Associate Lecturer, Veterinary Ophthalmology and Animal Welfare, Department
of Veterinary Medicine, University of Cambridge, Cambridge, United Kingdom

Contents

> In farm animal practice, there is often a clear tension between animal welfare and the economic basis of food animal production. Animal well-being is regularly compromised by the stringencies of intensive animal husbandry. Conditions such as infectious keratoconjunctivitis or ocular squamous cell carcinoma, while having negative effects on animal welfare, also have profoundly deleterious effects on animal production. This article discusses the welfare implications of the ocular conditions covered further in the following articles and how these affect treatment of these diseases.

> A step-wise procedure and necessary equipment for examination of the ruminant and camelid eye are detailed. Restraint techniques and usage of local anesthetics to facilitate examination are described. Common examination findings and their significance are discussed. Finally, therapeutic options for keratoconjunctivitis and uveitis are explored. A complete ocular examination of ruminants is often not performed in the field because of lack of time, lack of appropriate facilities, and/or lack of equipment. Although individual ophthalmic examinations are not frequently performed as part of a herd health program, they can be of value in select cases. Ocular manifestations of systemic diseases may assist the clinician in establishing a diagnosis on the farm and for little additional cost. For patients with a specific ocular complaint, a complete ophthalmic examination is critical. After completion of the examination and arrival at a diagnosis, one must also be cognizant of the therapeutic regimens that are appropriate for use in ruminants, particularly animals that may be used for meat or milk.

> Although many eye conditions can be managed medically, several require surgical intervention. This article aims to review those conditions with surgical treatment options before going on to consider the various aspects of surgery itself, whether that be in the field or in a hospital setting. Often the surgery one would ideally like to perform is limited by geographic issues of transporting the animal to a surgical facility, and thus attempts have to be

made to undertake the best operative procedures one can, given the field conditions available. Even more so, economic factors often limit the type of operations one would wish to carry out. Here, rather than reduce the surgical techniques discussed to the lowest common denominator, the author seeks to explore what is possible in the best situations, trusting that the reader can modify the operations described to fit the environment and animal they are faced with.

latitudes with higher levels of sunlight. Control of this disease would be of considerable significance to the economics and profitability of the beef and dairy cattle industries. This article reviews the characteristics of the most commonly affected animals, the factors that are believed to contribute to the development of OSCC, and the treatment options that have been proposed.

In the past 10 years, information about South American camelid anatomy, physiology, medicine, and surgery has increased exponentially, including information about the eye. Although trauma-related diseases are the most common eye problems for which camelids are presented to veterinarians, there have recently been many anecdotal reports and published case reports of camelids having ocular malignancies and potentially hereditary ocular abnormalities. The increased number of ocular diseases being reported may be because of increased recognition of camelid diseases or an increase in these diseases as a result of restricted gene pools as a consequence of inbreeding. As the popularity of camelids is steadily increasing, owners are becoming more knowledgeable about their animals, and there is more need for veterinarians who understand their ocular anatomy, physiology, disease susceptibility, and recommended treatments. This article provides the relevant information about the eye.

Although there appears to have been an increase in literature about the anatomy and physiology of the pig eye because of an expansion in its use as a model for research, there has been little written about the development of veterinary medicine in the area. Pig eyes share many similarities with human eyes, having a holangiotic retinal vasculature, no tapetum, cone photoreceptors in the outer retina, and a similar scleral thickness, rendering them valuable in comparative research. It must not be forgotten, however, that pigs are intelligent sentient animals which use vision as an important sense. Thus, diseases such as congenital cataracts, which impede vision, are important from the perspective of pig welfare. In addition, ocular lesions in this species, as with many others, can be a significant sign of systemic disease.

Bovine parainfluenza-3 virus (bPI$_3$V) is a long-recognized, currently underappreciated, endemic infection in cattle populations. Clinical disease is most common in calves with poor passive transfer or decayed maternal antibodies. It is usually mild, consisting of fever, nasal discharge, and dry cough. Caused at least partly by local immunosuppressive effects, bPI$_3$V infection is often complicated by coinfection with other respiratory viruses and bacteria, and is therefore an important component of enzootic pneumonia in calves and bovine respiratory disease complex in feedlot cattle. Active infection can be diagnosed by virus isolation from nasal swabs, or IF testing on smears made from nasal swabs. Timing of sampling is critical in obtaining definitive diagnostic test results. Parenteral and intranasal modified live vaccine combination vaccines are available. Priming early in calfhood with intranasal vaccine, followed by boosting with parenteral vaccine, may be the best immunoprophylactic approach.

RELATED INTEREST

Veterinary Clinics of North America: Small Animal Practice,
March 2008 (Vol. 38, no. 2)
Ophthalmic Immunology and Immune-mediated Disease
David L. Williams, MA, VetMB, PhD, CertVOphthal, FRCVS, *Guest Editor*

THE CLINICS ARE NOW AVAILABLE ONLINE!

Access your subscription at:
www.theclinics.com

Preface

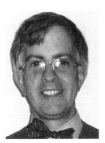

David L. Williams, MA, VetMB, PhD,
CertVOphthal, CertWEL, FRCVS
Guest Editor

When I had finished editing the *Veterinary Clinics of North America: Small Animal Practice* issue on Ophthalmic Immunology and Immune-mediated Disease in 2008, I was foolish enough to remark to the series editor what a shame it was that food animal ophthalmology had not been covered by the *Veterinary Clinics* series since 1984. There must be significant advances in the field, which would be worth documenting in a volume dedicated to the subject. I should have known that this comment would rebound on me with a request to edit just such an issue! I found it difficult to say no. There must have been a reason for this significant lacuna in the literature, and I was about to find out what that was! Large animal ophthalmology falls rather uncomfortably between two schools. Most veterinary ophthalmologists involve themselves predominantly in small animal, equine, or sometimes even exotic animal clinical work but rarely see a cow or sheep and even less frequently a pig. Most ocular disease in production animals is dealt with by farm animal veterinarians. There is simply not the economic wherewithal to involve a referral specialist in common conditions of ruminants and as such it is those first opinion veterinarians who have the most experience in ocular disease in these species. Thus it was not easy to find veterinarians who felt themselves suitably experienced in the practical aspects of the subjects on which I asked them to write and were prepared to devote the substantial resources in time and energy necessary to producing an article for this issue. It is thus with great thanks to the authors of articles within this volume that I present it to you. I trust that the information contained herein will be of value both to those who, as veterinary ophthalmologists, are not involved in a day-to-day manner with production animal eyes, and perhaps even more so to those who deal with them regularly, but often without the opportunity to read of new insights into diagnosis and treatment of conditions with which they are

Vet Clin Food Anim 26 (2010) xi–xii
doi:10.1016/j.cvfa.2010.09.005
0749-0720/10/$ – see front matter © 2010 Elsevier Inc. All rights reserved.

all too familiar at a practical level. We start with a tribute to one who has done so much for veterinary ophthalmology, and food animal ophthalmology particularly in his earlier years, Dr Keith Barnett, to which this volume is dedicated.

David L. Williams, MA, VetMB, PhD, CertVOphthal, CertWEL, FRCVS
Veterinary Ophthalmology and Animal Welfare
Department of Veterinary Medicine
University of Cambridge
Cambridge CB3 0ES, England, UK

E-mail addresses:
dlw33@cam.ac.uk
doctordlwilliams@aol.com

Tribute to Dr Keith Barnett

It seems entirely appropriate to dedicate this production animal ophthalmology issue of the *Veterinary Clinics of North America* to Dr Keith Barnett (**Fig. 1**), who, sadly, died in March 2009. Keith was born in his beloved Yorkshire in 1929 and knew he wanted to be a veterinarian from the age of five, living, as he did, in a house filled with animals. He studied at the Royal Veterinary College and after a period in general veterinary practice he worked as house surgeon in the Beaumont Animals' Hospital back at the RVC. There he came under the influence of Professor Gordon Knight and thus started his life-long passion for veterinary ophthalmology. He undertook his doctoral studies on progressive retinal atrophy in the dog there, which began a life's work on the subject, his name still appearing on research publications on the subject up until 2007. Indeed Keith's publication record is outstanding, with over 130 papers as well as enumerable articles and conference papers. Indeed there are only four years between 1965 and 2009 when his work did not appear somewhere in the published scientific literature! While most of these reports were in small animal ophthalmology, Dr Barnett made a significant impact on production animal ophthalmology. He published first in the large animal field on bright blindness in sheep (**Fig. 2**),[1,2] a retinopathy caused by ingestion of the toxin ptaquiloside from bracken (*Pteridium aquilinum*).[3]

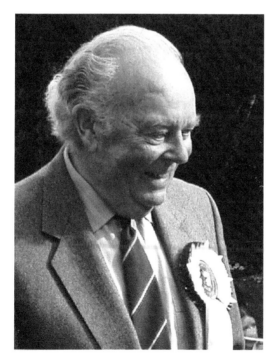

Fig. 1. Dr Keith Barnett, to whom this issue of *Veterinary Clinics* is dedicated. (*Courtesy* Animal Health Trust, Newmarket, UK.)

Vet Clin Food Anim 26 (2010) xiii–xvi
doi:10.1016/j.cvfa.2010.09.004   **vetfood.theclinics.com**
0749-0720/10/$ – see front matter © 2010 Elsevier Inc. All rights reserved.

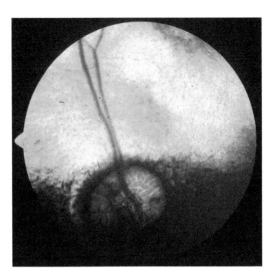

Fig. 2. Bright blindness in a bracken-fed sheep.

Dr Barnett's next published study was on the ocular effects of hypovitaminosis A in cattle,[4,5] with osteopathic effects on the skull foraminae leading to papilloedema and blindness. He left the Royal Veterinary College in London and joined the Department of Veterinary Clinical Studies in Cambridge where, with a Leverhulme Fellowship and support from the Animal Medical Center in New York, he started a Unit of Comparative Ophthalmology. 'Comparative' was a key word for Keith and, while his work on the dog and cat expanded continually, he was always interested in conditions in food animal ophthalmology, continuing his work on the sheep retina, collaborating with colleagues from Cambridge but also investigating conditions from optic nerve colobomas in Charolais cattle[6] to congenital cataracts in calves.[7] Keith always

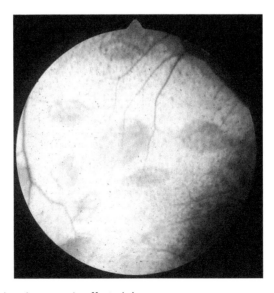

Fig. 3. Retinal lesions in a scrapie-affected sheep.

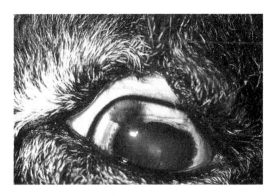

Fig. 4. Upper eyelid coloboma in one of Dr Barnett's four-horned Jacob sheep.

peppered his fascinating lectures with entertaining anecdotes, and one of my favorites was his story of covertly examining Charolais cattle in Dieppe Harbour, en route to England, to determine under cover of darkness which animals had the condition. He said that the French could never work out how the importers knew which animals were affected—I trust he will forgive me now for revealing his secret!

Dr Barnett was often way ahead of his time. He was the first to recognize retinal changes in sheep affected by scrapie[8] (**Fig. 3**) thirty years ahead of other's acceptance that ophthalmic evaluation can be a valuable diagnostic aid in prion diseases.[9]

But to Keith, there was always more to animals than merely their eyes, fascinating though those may be! He always enjoyed sheep and owned a flock of Soays and Jacobs (with upper eyelid colobomas associated with their four-horned-ness[10] (**Fig. 4**), animals that proved impossible to control. As Professor Sheila Crispin tells us in her obituary notice in an issue of *The Globe* dedicated to Keith's memory, "most people would have become annoyed and frustrated at the antics of this wayward flock but, quite remarkably, I cannot remember Keith ever becoming angry with anyone or anything; it was just not part of his nature."[11] Keith was always one who encouraged and enthused his colleagues and especially his juniors with a great passion for his chosen subject as well as his zest for life. As Sally Turner writes, "Each and every budding ophthalmologist who spent time with Keith became and remained a firm friend. And the fact that the vast majority went on to pursue careers in full time veterinary ophthalmology is a tribute to Keith's infectious dedication to our specialty."[10] As one of the many privileged to be able to count Keith as a mentor and friend, it is my pleasure to be able to dedicate this volume to his memory.

David L. Williams, MA, VetMB, PhD, CertVOphthal, CertWEL, FRCVS
Veterinary Ophthalmology and Animal Welfare
Department of Veterinary Medicine
University of Cambridge
Cambridge CB3 0ES, England, UK

E-mail address:
doctordlwilliams@aol.com

REFERENCES

1. Watson WA, Barlow RM, Barnett KC. Bright blindness—a condition prevalent in Yorkshire hill sheep. Vet Rec 1965;77:1060–9.

2. Barnett KC, Watson WA. Bright blindness in sheep—the results of further investigations. Veterinarian 1968;5:17—27.
3. Barnett KC, Watson WA. Bright blindness in sheep. A primary retinopathy due to feeding bracken (Pteris aquilina). Res Vet Sci 1970;11:289—90.
4. Abrams JT, Barnett KC, Bridge PS, et al. The retinol status and voluntary food consumption of the calf on a vitamin A-free diet. Int Z Vitaminforsch 1969;39: 416—25.
5. Barnett KC, Palmer AC, Abrams JT, et al. Ocular changes associated with hypovitaminosis A in cattle. Br Vet J 1970;126:561—73.
6. Barnett KC, Ogien AL. Ocular colobomata in Charolais cattle. Vet Rec 1972;91: 592.
7. Ashton, Barnett KC, Clay CE, et al. Congenital nuclear cataracts in cattle. Vet Rec 1977;100:505—8.
8. Barnett KC, Palmer AC. Retinopathy in sheep affected with natural scrapie. Res Vet Sci 1971;12:383—5.
9. Surguchev A, Surguchov A. Conformational diseases: looking into the eyes. Brain Res Bull 2010;81:12—24.
10. Henson EA. Study of the congenital defect 'split eyelid' in the multi-horned breeds of British sheep. Ark 1981;8:84—90.
11. The Globe, International Society for Veterinary Ophthalmology, April 2009. Available at: http://www.bravo.org.uk/THE%20GLOBE%20DEDICATED%20TO%20KEITH%20BARNETTpdf.pdf. Accessed September 8, 2010.

Welfare Issues in Farm Animal Ophthalmology

David L. Williams, MA, VetMB, PhD, CertVOphthal, CertWEL, FRCVS

KEYWORDS

• Eye disease • Farm animal welfare • Pain • Suffering

One of the most exciting days of my year as a university lecturer is the graduation ceremony for our students, the moment they become veterinarians. There and then the students affirm "my constant endeavor will be to ensure the welfare of the animals committed to my care."[1] Yet in farm animal practice, there is often a clear tension between animal welfare and the economic basis of food animal production.[2] It can be that animal welfare, animal well-being, is compromised by the stringencies of intensive animal husbandry. On the other hand, usually when disease impairs animal welfare, it also has deleterious effects on production. Conditions such as infectious keratoconjunctivitis or ocular squamous cell carcinoma, while having negative effects on animal welfare, also have profoundly deleterious effects on animal production.

In this article, the author discusses the welfare implications of the conditions covered in other articles in this issue and how these affect treatment of the diseases.

PAIN, SUFFERING, AND STRESS IN PRODUCTION ANIMALS

Pain may be defined as "an unpleasant sensory and emotional experience associated with actual or potential tissue damage, or described in terms of such damage"[3] While many from Descartes onwards considered that animals could not feel pain[4] or at least were not self-consciously aware of pain,[5] such a view is much less common today.[6] Given that animals, or at the very least mammals and birds, have the same nociceptive machinery as humans in terms of pain-related neurotransmitters, nociceptive neural pathways, and pain-sensing brain structures,[7] it would be foolish not to attribute somewhat similar pain sensations to them. These pain sensations account for the sensory aspect of the definition given earlier. What though of the emotional side of pain? Changes in behavior in animals exposed to painful stimuli show that response to a nociceptive stimulus is more than a mere reflex, yet the relationship between the injury itself and the response to pain can be varied and complex.[8] Indeed, a major part of the problem in assessing ocular pain in production animals, such as ruminants,

Veterinary Ophthalmology and Animal Welfare, Department of Veterinary Medicine, University of Cambridge, Cambridge CB3 0ES, England, UK
E-mail addresses: dlw33@cam.ac.uk; doctordlwilliams@aol.com

Vet Clin Food Anim 26 (2010) 427–435
doi:10.1016/j.cvfa.2010.08.005
0749-0720/10/$ – see front matter © 2010 Elsevier Inc. All rights reserved.

vetfood.theclinics.com

is that evolution has designed them to disguise much of their pain response. For example, lameness is a major problem in dairy cattle at present. Gait analysis shows that early signs of foot pain are missed by many farmers. Use of pedometers shows that changes in movement occur well before even the most assiduous cowman can detect obvious locomotor defects.[9] A survey of the available literature shows 718 articles on cattle lameness and 35 on the assessment of pain in these animals.

Yet, the only articles on ocular pain in ruminants concern the use of ex vivo bovine cornea models to assess ocular irritation[10] or changes in ocular temperature in calves subject to dehorning.[11] Although these topics are fascinating, it is deeply concerning that there is neither any literature on the pain experienced by cattle with an ocular disease, such as that illustrated in **Fig. 1**, nor on the importance (or indeed otherwise) of ameliorating such noxious stimuli.

Behavior changes in ruminants experiencing pain include separation from the flock or herd, decreased mutation exhibited as a reduced interest in surroundings and conspecifics, decreased appetite, bruxism (teeth grinding), dropping ears and head held below the withers, vocalization such as grunting either spontaneously or when the painful region is palpated, a hunched back and reluctance to move, restlessness, and in extreme situations, sternal or lateral recumbency with tachycardia.[12] Specific signs associated with ocular pain also include blepharospasm, epiphora, and guarding of the eye when approached. Yet, as noted earlier, many animals exhibit these signs to a far lesser degree than might be expected, given the pathology noted with corneal ulceration, intraocular inflammation, or periocular neoplastic change.

There is more to animal welfare than pain alone. The 5 freedoms approach to farm animal welfare originated from the Brambell Committee's report in 1965 in response to Harrison's[13] groundbreaking book *Animal Machines*. Modified a decade later by the Farm Animal Welfare Council (FAWC),[14] this strategy aims to identify basic freedoms from physiologic stress, pain, and suffering, which should be afforded to all animals under human care, as discussed in **Box 1**. Furthermore, a Universal Declaration on Animal Welfare proposed by the World Society for the Protection of Animals[15] calls on the United Nations to acknowledge animals as sentient beings, capable of experiencing pain and suffering, and to recognize animal welfare as an issue of importance as part of the social development internationally.

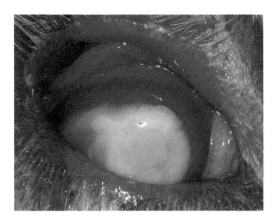

Fig. 1. Infectious bovine keratoconjunctivitis. Note the perilimbal hyperemic vascular fringe, the extensive corneal edema and ulceration, and the degree of epiphora demonstrating ocular surface pain.

> **Box 1**
> **The Farm Animal Welfare Council's 5 freedoms**
>
> - Freedom from thirst and hunger by providing ready access to fresh water and a diet to maintain full health and vigor.
> - Freedom from discomfort by providing an appropriate environment, including shelter and a comfortable resting area.
> - Freedom from pain, injury, and disease by prevention or rapid diagnosis and treatment.
> - Freedom to express normal behavior by providing sufficient space, proper facilities, and company of the animal's own kind.
> - Freedom from fear and distress by ensuring conditions and treatments that avoid mental suffering.

Freedom from pain, injury, and disease is clearly central to a veterinary approach to animal welfare and requires steps to minimize conditions resulting in noxious stimuli, but diseases that compromise vision have significant effects on the freedom to behavior normally and increase fear and distress. We should continually reflect on how these conditions are affecting all five of these freedoms (see **Box 1**).

INFECTIOUS BOVINE KERATOCONJUNCTIVITIS AND OCULAR SURFACE PAIN

Readers with a personal experience of corneal ulceration in their own eye will be able to testify to the extreme pain experienced from even a small erosion of the epithelial corneal surface, which is not surprising. The cornea is estimated to be the most densely innervated area of the body surface in each species investigated, from mice[16] to men.[17,18] There is no reason to think that ruminants should be any different, although the number of reports documenting bovine corneal innervation is vanishingly small.[19] Corneal nerves may be myelinated or nonmyelinated, though all end in nonmyelinated simple nerve endings without structural specialization of the ensheathing Schwann cells. Conduction velocity studies show these nerves to be C-fiber or A delta axons, both known to be involved in pain sensation in other organisms. So, these free nerve endings of corneal nerves give a sensation of pain, whatever the stimulus,[20] although this function has been debated for some years. Lele and Weddell[21] reported that touch, warmth, and cold could be detected as well as pain, whereas Beuerman and colleagues[22,23] found that any noxious sensation was felt as irritation and pain only if the cornea was stimulated.

Corneal injuries provoke some degree of breakdown in the blood-aqueous barrier and the generation of a uveitic reponse,[24] with this change being mediated by trigeminal stimulation mediated predominantly, but not entirely, by a prostaglandin-mediated pathway.[25] Thus ocular surface inflammation is not only provoked by corneal damage, physical, chemical, or, as in the case of infectious bovine keratoconjunctivitis (IBK), biologic agents. Intraocular inflammation does not require the inciting agent to enter the globe but can be brought about by these neural and biochemical pathways. The resulting muscular spasms bring about much of the ocular pain in uveitis and keratouveitis (see later discussion on listerial uveitis and keratouveitic pain).

Given all this information, the noxious stimulus apprehended when the cornea is damaged in a case such as that illustrated in **Fig. 1**, a cow with acute IBK, must be significant. No wonder IBK often results in a dull depressed animal with impeded appetitive behaviors and a reduced weight gain. However, in an ongoing study, as yet unpublished, the author has found that it can be difficult to quantify abnormal behaviors in chronically affected animals because diseased cattle generally masked signs suggestive of pain and discomfort. Such obscuration of pain is a common feature in prey species because predators target animals in distress. The same problems occur in laboratory rodent species in which telemetric evaluation of heart rate and heart rate variability are two of the few methods of assessing postoperative pain.[26] A more concrete approach to determining pain responses to corneal injury as seen in IBK is needed; indeed, a key part of this article is not only to look back at work in the past but also to suggest areas for future study. One such area is described.

LISTERIAL UVEITIS AND KERATOUVEITIC PAIN

The classic features of any inflammation are rubor, calor, tumor, and dolor, that is, redness, heat, swelling, and pain. An inflamed eye with keratitis, uveitis, or a combination of both as in many cases of silage eye (**Fig. 2**) exhibits increased vascular congestion, inflammatory cell proliferation, and spasm of the iridal and ciliary muscles with miosis and ciliary body–derived pain. Another associated noxious stimulus is photophobia, the intolerance to bright light. Understanding these features of the response to uveitis helps to control it better. It is ironic that given that photophobia has been recognized as a severe ocular disability for years,[27] it is only in 2010 that the neurologic link between bright light and noxious trigeminal stimulation has been proved,[28] This link explains why topical nonsteroidal medication can be so beneficial in photophobia.[29–31]

However, the pain in intraocular inflammation, in uveitis, is not generated solely by this light-related mechanism. The iridal spasm, which results in miosis with the pupil tightly closed, also affects the muscles of the ciliary body, just posterior to the iris root. It is probably this iridociliary spasm, which causes most pain in uveitis, meaning that the use of a cycloplegic, such as atropine, is to be welcomed in any such case. It is difficult, of course, to define what proportion of the ocular analgesic effect of

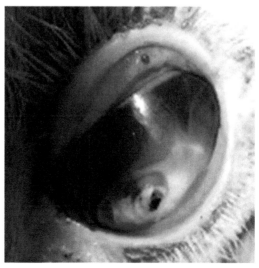

Fig. 2. Silage eye in an alpaca with keratitis and uveitis. (*Courtesy of* Dr J. D. Lavach, Reno, NV.)

antiuveitic medication is owed to the spasmolytic effects of atropine because treatment of such intraocular inflammation should include cycloplegia concurrent with antiinflammatory medication. It is known that there are nociceptive nerve endings in the iris itself,[32] although the influence of these on pain in intraocular inflammation is unclear. Topical and systemic nonsteroidals themselves have analgesic effects,[33] but of course the search is for a multimodal therapeutic approach to pain control wherever it is directed, so such opportunities for using several different agents is theoretically to be welcomed.[34]

Control of the inflammation is clearly vital. Yet there is a problem. If the etiologic agent is infectious, as would seem to be the case in most cases of silage eye, should steroidal or nonsteroidal antiinflammatory agents be used in the face of bacterial or maybe even viral infection? The important features of all such treatments are the reduction in pain and restoration or maintenance of vision. In this area we might consider ourselves fortunate. Physicians face the problem that long-term steroid treatment, while reducing the inflammation, also has the side effect of steroid-induced glaucoma or steroid-induced cataract in many people. While cattle can be provoked to raised intraocular pressure by prolonged use of steroid,[35] with ultrastructural extracellular matrix changes[36] similar to those seen in people with steroid-induced glaucoma,[37] a cost-benefit analysis shows that reducing the inflammation is vital in such cases and as such topical or subconjunctival steroids are the preferred treatment option.

OCULAR SQUAMOUS CELL CARCINOMA AND ADNEXAL PAIN

Squamous cell carcinoma affecting the eye is a major cause of carcase condemnation and as such a significant financial burden to farmers in areas where the disease is common.[38,39] Yet underlying these economic facts is a significant welfare implication with cows, such as the one shown in **Fig. 3**, having significant morbidity. The epiphora, ocular discharge, and self-trauma point to substantial effects from discomfort to frank pain. Yet these effects on animal welfare are rarely, if ever, alluded to in reports of the condition. Treatment regimes, from bacille Calmette-Guérin immunotherapy to enucleation, may resolve this pain and discomfort, but given that many of these animals are out at pasture long-term and may not be seen until the lesion is extensive

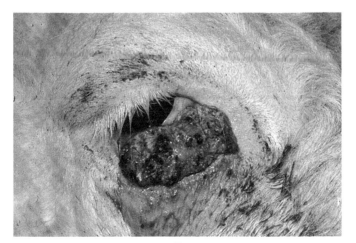

Fig. 3. Advanced bovine ocular squamous cell carcinoma.

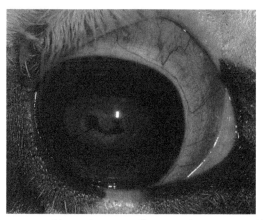

Fig. 4. Congenital cataract with persistent pupillary membranes in a calf.

and already causing welfare problems, efforts to use cattle less prone to the condition is important.

CONGENITAL CATARACT AND BLINDNESS

In all of this the welfare implications of blindness and visual compromise have not been considered. What of animals affected with disorders such as nuclear cataract, which affects their vision (**Fig. 4**). In several studies, a considerable minority of calves were affected by nuclear cataract, with effects on vision in up to a quarter of animals.[40,41] Although it might be argued that ruminants have less of an absolute requirement for excellent vision than do other species groups, such as the carnivores and more specifically humans, a profound effect on vision cannot be a positive influence on an animal's health and welfare.

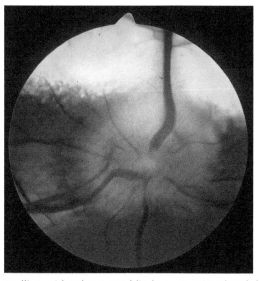

Fig. 5. Optic nerve swelling with subsequent blindness associated with hypovitaminosis A.

Turning back to the FAWC's five freedoms considered earlier, visual compromise may affect freedom from hunger and thirst if an animal is less able to reach feeding and water stations. Equally, blind animals are less able to fulfill normal behaviors and likely to have increased levels of fear and distress. But there is a frustrating lack of concrete evidence on these matters. Levels of stress, as documented by increased levels of circulating stress hormones such as cortisol, have yet to be determined in animals with ocular lesions causing blindness or ocular pain. How much are blind calves with nuclear cataracts or the optic neuropathy of hypovitaminosis A (**Fig. 5**) really affected by their disability?

More research is clearly needed on the effects of visual compromise on the welfare of farm animals. Indeed, the effect on animal welfare of low light levels in intensive poultry production systems and the suggestion that genetically blind chickens could be used to reduce deleterious interactions between birds in high-density rearing systems have not been discussed.[42] It is to be hoped that the articles in this issue will stimulate more research in these areas.

SUMMARY

It might be considered unusual to start an issue focusing on large animal ophthalmology with a contribution on animal welfare. As has been noted earlier, affective disorders associated with ocular pain and discomfort or visual compromise in food-producing animals are rarely considered when discussing conditions such as corneal ulceration, uveitis, or ocular neoplasia. But the author admits that the same might be said of companion animal and equine ophthalmology. Woefully little attention is paid to ocular pain when it does not stare us in the face. Much research is still needed in identifying and treating ocular pain and discomfort in all animal species, but perhaps particularly in these food-producing animals, which, as prey species, tend, as we have discussed earlier, to mask their discomfort. The fact that these animals do not manifest such signs does not indicate that the pain does not exist but that we need to be more assiduous in identifying when it might be present. Similarly, a better understanding of the effect of visual dysfunction on the welfare of any animal but particularly those kept for milk, meat, or fiber is needed.

REFERENCES

1. Hewson CJ. Veterinarians who swear: animal welfare and the veterinary oath. Can Vet J 2006;47:807–11.
2. Webster AJ. Farm animal welfare: the five freedoms and the free market. Vet J 2001;161:229–37.
3. Bonica JJ. "The need of a taxonomy." Pain 1979;6(3):247–52, this definition in humans was originally penned by Merskey, H (1964). An Investigation of pain in psychological illness, DM Thesis. Oxford University.
4. Bermond B. The myth of animal suffering. In: Dol M, Kasanmoentalib S, Lijmbach S, et al, editors. Animal consciousness and animal ethics. The Netherlands: Van Gorcum Publishers; 1997. p. 153–67.
5. Cottingham John. "'A brute to the brutes'? Descartes' treatment of animals,". Philosophy 1988;63:175–83.
6. Bateson P. Assessment of pain in animals. Anim Behav 1991;42:827–39.
7. Short CE. Fundamentals of pain perception in animals. Appl Anim Behav Sci 1998;59:125–33.
8. Wall PD. On the relation of injury to pain. The John J. Bonica lecture. Pain 1979;6:253–64.

9. Mazrier H, Tal S, Aizinbud E, et al. A field investigation of the use of the pedometer for the early detection of lameness in cattle. Can Vet J 2006;47:883–6.

10. Cater KC, Harbell JW. Comparison of in vitro eye irritation potential by bovine corneal opacity and permeability (BCOP) assay to erythema scores in human eye sting test of surfactant-based formulations. Cutan Ocul Toxicol 2008;27:77–85.

11. Stewart M, Stafford KJ, Dowling SK, et al. Eye temperature and heart rate variability of calves disbudded with or without local anaesthetic. Physiol Behav 2008;93:789–97.

12. Flecknell PA, Waterman A. Pain management in animals. London: WB Saunders; 2000.

13. Harrison R. Animal machines: the new factory farming industry. London: Vincent Stuart; 1964. p. 186.

14. Available at: http://www.fawc.org.uk/freedoms.htm. Accessed September 20, 2010.

15. Available at: http://www.wspa.org.uk/animalsmatter/UDAWText2005.pdf. Accessed September 20, 2010.

16. Yu CQ, Rosenblatt MI. Transgenic corneal neurofluorescence in mice: a new model for in vivo investigation of nerve structure and regeneration. Invest Ophthalmol Vis Sci 2007;48:1535–42.

17. Marfurt CF, Cox J, Deek S, et al. Anatomy of the human corneal innervation. Exp Eye Res 2010;90:478–92.

18. Müller LJ, Vrensen GF, Pels L, et al. Architecture of human corneal nerves. Invest Ophthalmol Vis Sci 1997;38:985–94.

19. Osborne NN. The occurrence of serotonergic nerves in the bovine cornea. Neurosci Lett 1983;35:15–8.

20. Matthews B. Peripheral and central aspects of trigeminal nociceptive systems. Philos Trans R Soc Lond B Biol Sci 1985;308(1136):313–24.

21. Lele PP, Weddell G. Sensory nerves of the cornea and cutaneous sensibility. Exp Neurol 1959;1:334–59.

22. Beuerman RW, Snow A, Thompson H, et al. Action potential response of the corneal nerves to irritants. Lens Eye Toxic Res 1992;9(3–4):193–210.

23. Beuerman RW, Tanelian DL. Corneal pain evoked by thermal stimulation. Pain 1979;7:1–14.

24. Jampol LM, Neufeld AH, Sears ML. Pathways for the response of the eye to injury. Invest Ophthalmol 1975;14:184–9.

25. Eakins KE. Prostaglandin and non-prostaglandin mediated breakdown of the blood-aqueous barrier. Exp Eye Res 1977;25(Suppl):483–98.

26. Arras M, Rettich A, Cinelli P, et al. Assessment of post-laparotomy pain in laboratory mice by telemetric recording of heart rate and heart rate variability. BMC Vet Res 2007;3:16.

27. Göbel H, Isler H, Hasenfratz HP. Headache classification and the Bible: was St Paul's thorn in the flesh migraine? Cephalalgia 1995;15:180–1.

28. Okamoto K, Tashiro A, Chang Z, et al. Bright light activates a trigeminal nociceptive pathway. Pain 2010;149:235–42.

29. Kim SJ, Flach AJ, Jampol LM. Nonsteroidal anti-inflammatory drugs in ophthalmology. Surv Ophthalmol 2010;55:108–33.

30. Giuliano EA. Nonsteroidal anti-inflammatory drugs in veterinary ophthalmology. Vet Clin North Am Small Anim Pract 2004;34:707–23.

31. Chitkara DK, Jayamanne DG, Griffiths PG, et al. Effectiveness of topical diclofenac in relieving photophobia after pupil dilation. J Cataract Refract Surg 1997;23:740–4.

32. Lehtosalo JI, Uusitalo H, Palkama A. Sensory supply of the anterior uvea: a light and electron microscope study. Exp Brain Res 1984;55:562–9.
33. Chen X, Gallar J, Belmonte C. Reduction by antiinflammatory drugs of the response of corneal sensory nerve fibers to chemical irritation. Invest Ophthalmol Vis Sci 1997;38:1944–53.
34. Lamont LA. Multimodal pain management in veterinary medicine: the physiologic basis of pharmacologic therapies. Vet Clin North Am Small Anim Pract 2008;38: 1173–86.
35. Gerometta R, Podos SM, Candia OA, et al. Steroid-induced ocular hypertension in normal cattle. Arch Ophthalmol 2004;122:1492–7.
36. Tektas OY, Hammer CM, Danias J, et al. Morphologic changes in the outflow pathways of bovine eyes treated with corticosteroids. Invest Ophthalmol Vis Sci 2010;51:4060–6.
37. Johnson D, Gottanka J, Flügel C, et al. Ultrastructural changes in the trabecular meshwork of human eyes treated with corticosteroids. Arch Ophthalmol 1997; 115:375–83.
38. Grahn BH, Wolfer J. Canadian condemnation rate for bovine ocular squamous cell carcinoma. Can Vet J 1994;35:133.
39. Heeney JL, Valli VE. Bovine ocular squamous cell carcinoma: an epidemiological perspective. Can J Comp Med 1985;49:21–6.
40. Hässig M, Jud F, Naegeli H, et al. Prevalence of nuclear cataract in Swiss veal calves and its possible association with mobile telephone antenna base stations. Schweiz Arch Tierheilkd 2009;151:471–8.
41. Ashton NA, Barnett KC, Clay CE, et al. Congenital nuclear cataracts in cattle. Vet Rec 1977;100:505–8.
42. Thompson PB. The opposite of human enhancement: nanotechnology and the blind chicken problem. Nanoethics 2008;2:305–16.

Examination Techniques and Therapeutic Regimens for the Ruminant and Camelid Eye

Wendy M. Townsend, DVM, MS*

KEYWORDS

• Ruminant • Camelid • Eye • Ocular • Examination • Therapy

EXAMINATION

A systemic assessment of the visual system is critical. Use of a standardized examination sheet ensures that no critical steps are inadvertently missed (**Fig. 1**).

Restraint

Particularly when dealing with cattle, proper restraint of the patient is critical both for the examiner's safety and to complete a detailed examination. Sheep and goats can be backed into a corner and their head restrained by an assistant. Sheep can also be tipped so they are sitting on their rump. A sheep trimming/blocking stand or goat milking stand is very useful, as it elevates the animal to a more comfortable working position for the examiner and restrains the animal's head. Camelids can be restrained with either a halter or lead rope, or may be placed within a grooming chute. If the camelid is particularly fractious, placing a towel through the noseband of the halter so that it drapes over the muzzle can protect one from being spat upon (**Fig. 2**). Dairy cattle may be examined in a stanchion or head catch. Beef cattle are best examined within a head catch and squeeze chute. In addition, placement of nose tongs or a halter and rope lead to pull the head laterally and secure it can greatly facilitate completion of the examination (**Fig. 3**). Fractious animals may require the administration of a sedative agent. Remember that the use of α2-adrenergic agonists in ruminants can cause abortion late in pregnancy.[1] See **Table 1** for suggested sedation protocols and withdrawal intervals (WDI) within the United States.

The authors have nothing to disclose.

Comparative Ophthalmology, Department of Small Animal Clinical Sciences, Michigan State University, D208 Veterinary Medical Center, East Lansing, MI 48824-1314, USA

* School of Veterinary Medicine, Purdue University, 625 Harrison Street, West Lafayette, IN 47909-2026.

E-mail address: townsenw@purdue.edu

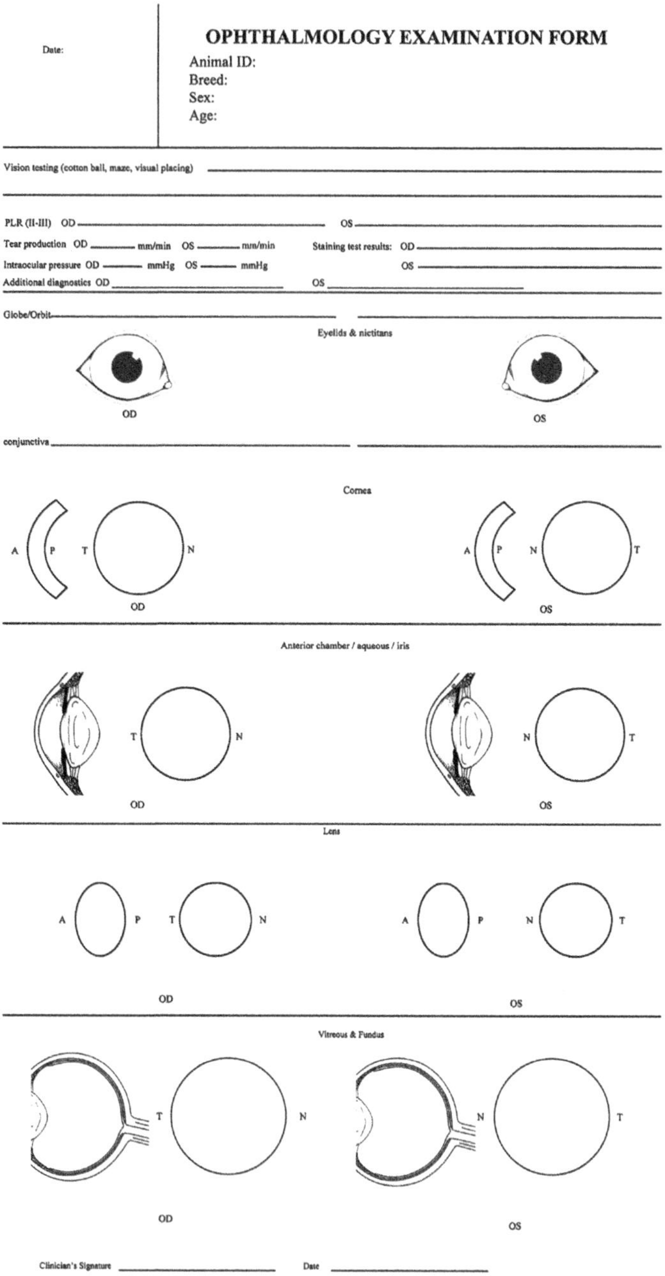

Fig. 1. Sample examination sheet.

Akinesia and Local Anesthesia

If the animal is extremely painful or if local manipulations are required, akinesia of the eyelids and local anesthesia of the affected area may facilitate examination. Topical anesthesia of the cornea and conjunctival surface may be achieved through instillation of

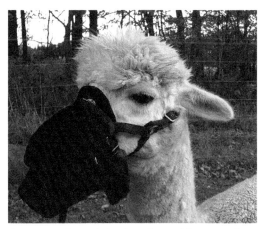

Fig. 2. Use of a towel to preventing spitting by a llama. (*Courtesy of* Dr Matthew Townsend, DVM, Dirigo Alpacas, Waterville, ME.)

a topical ocular anesthetic such as 1% proparacaine hydrochloride. After instillation of 1 to 2 drops, the cornea typically remains anesthetized for 10 to 20 minutes. As the conjunctiva is vascularized, local anesthesia is more difficult to obtain and lasts for a shorter period of time. Application of several drops and then holding a cotton swab soaked in the topical anesthetic on the area of interest will improve the degree of anesthesia obtained.

To facilitate opening of the eyelids, local anesthetics (eg, lidocaine hydrochloride injectable solution) can be infiltrated around the auriculopalpebral nerve. The nerve can be palpated as it crosses the zygomatic arch. Insert a 25-gauge needle in smaller ruminants. In adult cattle, especially bulls, one may need a heavier-gauge needle to penetrate the skin. Then attach a syringe containing the local anesthetic and infiltrate 1 to 2 mL (**Fig. 4**). One should limit the total dosage of lidocaine infused to 6 mg/kg.[2] One must be particularly careful in lambs and kids because of their small body sizes. Dilution of the lidocaine with saline to a 0.5% solution will allow for sufficient volume for injection without exceeding a safe systemic dose in smaller ruminants. When using local anesthetics, a meat and milk WDI of 24 hours is recommended.[3]

Assessment of Vision

Initial clues that a ruminant is having difficulties with vision are often gained by observing the animal within its environment. Visually impaired animals may be more

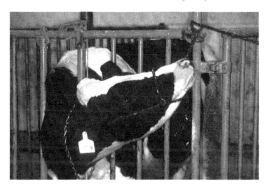

Fig. 3. Cow restrained for examination.

Table 1
Suggested sedation protocols and withdrawal intervals within the United States

Species	Drug Dosage	Withdrawal Interval in the USA
Cattle	0.01–0.03 mg/kg IV or 0.05 mg/kg IM of xylazine for sedation without recumbency[50]	4 d for meat and 24 h for milk[51]
Sheep	100–200 μg/kg IV or 200–400 μg/kg IM of xylazine[2]	5 d for meat and 72 h for milk after IV injection; 10 d for meat and 120 h for milk after IM injection[46]
Goats	50 μg/kg IV or 100 μg/kg IM of xylazine[2]	5 d for meat and 72 h for milk after IV injection; 10 d for meat and 120 h for milk after IM injection[46]
Camelids	0.1–0.2 mg/kg xylazine IV or 0.1 mg/kg xylazine + 0.05–0.1 mg/kg butorphanol IM[52]	

Abbreviations: IM, intramuscular; IV, intravenous.

easily startled, may run into other animals and objects, may be hesitant to move, and may fail to stay with the herd. The animal's behavior as it is caught for examination may also provide clues regarding the degree and location of the visual impairment. Because of the lateral position of their globes, ruminants have a wide field of vision. When a person enters their flight zone they should move, raise their heads, or otherwise indicate that the person was visualized. Failure to do so may indicate visual impairment. Once the animal is restrained, one may move the hand in a menacing gesture toward the eye (**Fig. 5**). The animal should turn its head away, retract the globe, or blink in response. The examiner must be cautious to avoid touching the eyelashes or vibrissae, which could also stimulate a blink response. Large hand movements may create air currents that stimulate false-positive responses as the animal detects the air movement across its cornea.

If the animal appears visual and yet fails to blink, one must ensure that the individual is capable of blinking. Touching the periocular skin both nasally and temporally should stimulate a blink through the palpebral reflex (**Fig. 6**). Failure to blink indicates either a deficit in sensation (cranial nerve V = trigeminal nerve: ophthalmic branch nasally

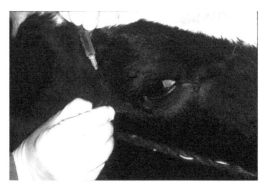

Fig. 4. Performing an auriculopalpebral nerve block. The skin is tented and the needle is inserted parallel to the surface of the underlying zygomatic arch. One to 1.5 mL of local anesthetic is then infiltrated.

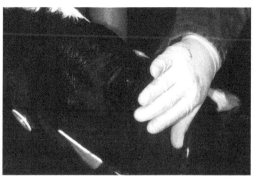

Fig. 5. Checking the menace response. The hand is moved in front of the eye taking care to avoid creating air currents or touching vibrissae.

and maxillary branch temporally) or a deficit in motor innervation (cranial nerve VII = facial nerve). Due to its superficial position, trauma to the side of the head may compromise the facial nerve. Such injuries may occur in cattle as the head catch is being closed if they back up or fail to place their head completely through the opening. Infection with *Listeria monocytogenes* may also cause cranial nerve deficits, including loss of the palpebral reflex through facial nerve paralysis at the level of the brainstem.[4]

Pupil Size and Pupillary Light Reflex

The ruminant pupil is an oval with the axis oriented horizontally. Spherical, black masses are present along the pupil's dorsal edge with smaller, similarly shaped masses ventrally (**Fig. 7**). These masses are called corpora nigra or granula iridica, and augment the effectiveness of pupillary constriction.[5] The masses are extensions of the posterior pigmented iridal epithelium. In camelids, a similar structure, the pupillary rough, presents as a pleated ruffle along the pupil's dorsal and ventral edges.

The pupil size and pupillary light reflex (PLR) should be assessed using a focal light source such as a Finnoff transilluminator (**Fig. 8**) or penlight with halogen bulb. Darkening the examination area greatly facilitates this portion of the examination. The pupils should be of equal size, symmetrically shaped, and appropriately sized for the ambient lighting conditions: relatively mydriatic (dilated) in the dark and relatively miotic (constricted) in bright light. As light is directed into the eye, the pupil should

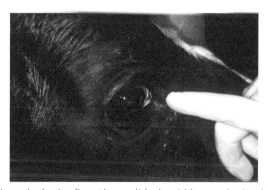

Fig. 6. Checking the palpebral reflex. The eyelids should be touched at both the inner and outer canthi to ensure appropriate sensation and the ability to blink.

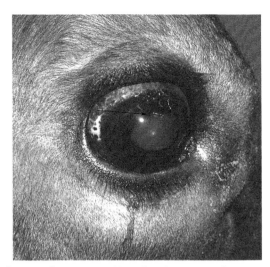

Fig. 7. Normal bovine anterior segment. Note the glossy, smooth appearance of the cornea. Note also the horizontal elliptical shape of the pupil and the presence of granula iridica (*arrow*).

constrict (the direct PLR). At the same time, the contralateral pupil should constrict (the indirect or consensual PLR). However, the high percentage of fibers that decussate at the optic chiasm (80%–90% in large animals) cause the indirect PLR to be slower and less complete than the direct PLR.[6]

It is important to remember that the PLR is not a test of vision. If the animal is blind and the PLR is absent, then the lesion is located within the retina, optic nerve, optic chiasm, or early portions of the optic tract. Possible causes include vitamin A deficiency, thromboembolic meningoencephalitis (*Histophilus somnus*) infection with retinal detachment and intraretinal hemorrhages, male fern (*Dryopteris filix-mas*) poisoning, bracken fern (*Pteridium aquilinum*) poisoning, and locoweed poisoning.[4] If the animal is blind and the PLR is intact, then the lesion must be located centrally within the visual cortex. Possible causes include lead toxicity,[7] polioencephalomalacia,[8] water deprivation/sodium ion toxicosis,[9] thromboembolic meningoencephalitis (*Histophilus somnus*) infection with multifocal hemorrhage and necrosis within the brain,[10] ketosis, and hypoglycemia.

Orbit and Globe

The size of the globe and its position within the orbit should be assessed. Congenital abnormalities include microphthalmos, which may be so marked as to mimic anophthalmos (complete absence of the eye) and cyclopia or synophthalmos (fusing of the globes). Calves infected with bovine virus diarrhea (BVD) between days 76 and 150 of gestation may be born with microphthalmos.[11] Persistently infected calves have also

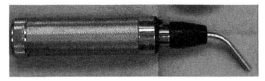

Fig. 8. Finnoff transilluminator.

been noted to have narrow skulls with bulging eyes.[12] Cyclopia in lambs may result if the ewe ingests *Veratrum californicum* (skunk cabbage) on day 14 of gestation.[13]

The globe may become enlarged (buphthalmic) due to chronic glaucoma or intraocular neoplasia. A markedly buphthalmic eye may preclude closing of the eyelids, leading to exposure keratitis and corneal ulceration. Most animals with buphthalmic globes are permanently blind in the affected eye. Therefore, enucleation is recommended if the animal is to remain in the herd or flock to remove discomfort associated with chronic elevations in intraocular pressure and any resultant exposure keratitis. Buphthalmos and exophthalmos (protrusion of the globe from the orbit) can sometimes cause diagnostic confusion as a markedly enlarged globe will also begin to protrude from the orbit. One can use measurement of the horizontal corneal diameter to differentiate the 2 lesions. If one compares the corneal diameter of the affected globe with the contralateral, unaffected globe and the affected globe has a larger diameter, then the eye is buphthalmic. If the affected and unaffected globes are equal, then the globe is exophthalmic.

Unilateral exophthalmos or strabismus (ocular misalignment) usually results from space-occupying lesions caused by inflammation or neoplasia. Increased resistance on retropulsion of the globe confirms the presence of a space-occupying lesion (**Fig. 9**). In cattle, lymphosarcoma affecting the retrobulbar tissues is the most frequent cause of exophthalmos (**Fig. 10**).[14] Squamous cell carcinoma may also extend into the orbit from the nasal cavity or periocular tissues. Exophthalmos may also result from chronic frontal sinusitis either subsequent to dehorning or associated with respiratory tract disease.[15] Dairy cattle, particularly Holstein, Ayrshire, Jersey, and German Brown Swiss, may exhibit a bilateral convergent strabismus (cross-eyes) with exophthalmia.[14] The lesion may progress until the animal reaches maturity and then stabilize. Although vision may be compromised, the animals appear to function normally within a herd. A genetic basis is suspected. The globe may also be enophthalmic or recessed within the orbit. Enophthalmos is seen most often in association with ocular pain.

Nystagmus (involuntary rapid movement of the eyeball) may be noted as a congenital finding, particularly in Holstein cattle.[16] Nystagmus may also occur in animals with congenital blindness. A ventrolateral or ventromedial strabismus or vertical or horizontal nystagmus may be noted in patients with listeriosis (**Fig. 11**).[17] Malignant catarrhal fever can cause nystagmus in association with the "head and eye" form of the disease.[18] Rabies can also cause nystagmus as a portion of the ocular manifestations, and therefore should be considered as a differential if this clinical sign is noted.[4]

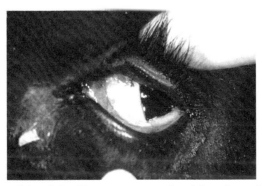

Fig. 9. Retropulsion of the globe. Place pressure on the globe using a finger on the upper eyelid. The globe should retropulse easily and the third eyelid should elevate.

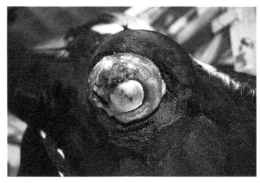

Fig. 10. Marked exophthalmos due to orbital lymphosarcoma in a Holstein cow. The exophthalmos is causing exposure keratitis as the cow can no longer blink over the cornea.

Variable nystagmus and a dorsomedial strabismus are often noted in cases of polioencephalomalacia.[8]

Eyelids

The entirety of the eyelids should be examined. Eyelid position should be noted. The lid margin should be smooth with a distinct haired/nonhaired junction. Particular attention should be paid to irregularities in the eyelid margin that may prevent normal dispersion of the tear-film, and eyelid ulcerations that may signify the presence of squamous cell carcinoma. The eyelids should be everted for inspection of the palpebral conjunctiva. The eyelids should be freely moveable and should close in response to digital pressure both medially and laterally. A negative palpebral reflex indicates loss of sensation (cranial nerve V), loss of motor innervation (cranial nerve VII), or a physical barrier to closure. In cattle, sheep, and goats, meibomian gland duct openings are noted along both the upper and lower eyelid margins. Camelids do not possess meibomian glands.[19]

Inversion of the eyelid margin, entropion, can occur in all ruminants (**Fig. 12**), predominantly as a congenital lesion. In sheep, entropion is relatively common with a reported incidence of 1.0% to 80.0%.[20–23] The resultant trichiasis may lead to corneal ulceration, vascularization, and scarring. Treatment involves eversion of the

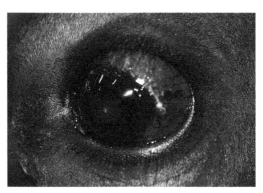

Fig. 11. Medial strabismus in a Jersey cow.

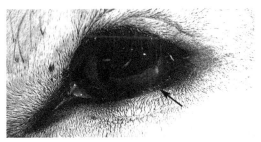

Fig. 12. Lower eyelid entropion in a year old Piedmont heifer. Note the resultant trichiasis (*arrow*).

affected eyelid. Ectropion, or rolling out of the eyelid margin, is rare, but has also been reported in cattle, sheep, and camelids.

In ruminants, blepharitis or inflammation of the eyelids is most often due to an infectious dermatitis or photosensitization. Dermatophilosis (rain scald, lumpy wool) affects all ruminants and causes painful lesions composed of proliferative, suppurative crusts and matted hair.[24] Although the muzzle is more often affected, in severe cases it may spread over the entire face.[25] Diagnosis is facilitated by cytologic examination of the suppurative exudates to visualize the characteristic "railroad appearance" of the organisms.[24] Dermatophytosis (ringworm) is common in cattle and relatively rare in sheep and goats.[26] The periocular region is frequently involved in cattle and the lesions are characterized by multifocal alopecia, scaling, and crusting, which can be excessive and take on a wart-like appearance.[26] The main differential diagnosis is dermatophilosis. Fungal cultures are the best method for diagnosis.[26]

In sheep and goats, secondary infection with *Actinobacillus lignieresii* may cause the formation of pyogranulomatous nodules with draining tracts.[27] Sarcoptic mange may cause thick, crusted, and denuded areas around the eyelids with an intense pruritus.[28] This condition is reportable within the United States. Demodectic mange may cause formation of pustules and abscess, which may or may not be pruritic.[28] Pox viruses and orbivirus (Blue tongue) may cause lesions in sheep and goats.[27] In camelids, blepharitis is most often associated with bacterial conjunctivitis, so close examination of the conjunctiva is warranted.

Photosensitization may occur due to ingestion of a photodynamic agent (primary photosensitization) or accumulation of phylloerythrin due to hepatitis or biliary duct obstruction (secondary photosensitization).[28] Photodynamic agents include hypericin in St John's wort, fagopyrin in buckwheat, perloline from perennial ryegrass, and phenothiazine sulfoxide from phenothiazine.[28,29] Photosensitization is characterized by erythema, edema, pruritus, necrosis, and sloughing of nonpigmented skin.[30] Removing the affected animal from direct sunlight and preventing ingestion of the offending agent are critical goals of therapy.

Nasolacrimal System

Normal secretions from the lacrimal glands should create a moist, glistening ocular surface. If the ocular surface appears dry, aqueous tear production may be assessed through the placement of a Schirmer tear test strip in the lower lateral conjunctival fornix for 1 minute. Tear production must be assessed before any agents have been instilled in the eye to prevent falsely elevated values. Normal readings are greater than 20 mm per minute.[31] The upper and lower puncta as well as the nasal opening of the nasolacrimal duct must be identified. Epiphora or overflow of tears onto the face should be noted if present. One should look for the presence of conjunctival foreign bodies, environmental irritants, conjunctivitis, corneal ulceration, or uveitis, which increase tear production, or atresias (acquired obstructions of the nasolacrimal apparatus), which prevent the flow of tears. Congenital abnormalities of the nasolacrimal system appear to be relatively common among the camelids.[32]

To assess patency of the nasolacrimal system, one may instill fluorescein dye into the conjunctival fornix and then monitor for its appearance at the nasal puncta within 5 to 20 minutes after instillation (Jones test) (**Fig. 13**). A negative test suggests the presence of an obstruction within the nasolacrimal system. Irrigation should be performed either retrograde (from the opening within the nares) or normograde (from the eyelid puncta). One should apply topical anesthetic (proparacaine ophthalmic solution to the eye or lidocaine gel to the nares) first, then cannulate the orifice using an open-ended tomcat catheter, 5F feeding tube, 4F to 6F polyethylene urinary catheter, teat cannula, or lacrimal cannula (normograde approach). Attach a 12- to 20-mL syringe filled with eyewash or saline solution and gently irrigate the nasolacrimal system until fluids exits. Digital pressure over the cannulated orifice may be required to prevent the backflush of fluid. Excessive force should be avoided. If the nasolacrimal system cannot be flushed, then skull radiographs, computed tomography or magnetic resonance imaging, and a contrast dye study would be indicated.

Conjunctiva

Darkening the examination area will facilitate the remainder of the ocular examination. The third eyelid, bulbar, and palpebral conjunctiva should be examined using focused illumination. Normal conjunctiva appears moist, semitransparent, and freely movable. The conjunctiva may become hyperemic with inflammation, pale with anemia, or yellow with icterus. Note the presence and character of any ocular discharge. The conjunctival sac should be examined for the presence of foreign bodies or nematodes (*Thelazia* sp).[33] Specific attention must be paid to areas of conjunctiva that appear raised, thickened, edematous (chemotic), ulcerated, or adherent, demonstrate follicle formation (cobblestoned appearance), have altered pigmentation, or exhibit mass lesions. The color and contour of the underlying sclera should be noted. The position

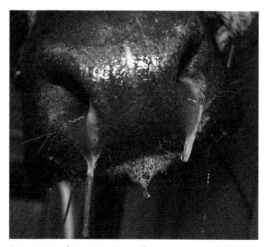

Fig. 13. A positive Jones test demonstrating the presence of fluorescein dye within the nares.

of the third eyelid and appearance of the free margin should be examined. After application of a topical anesthetic, the free margin of the third eyelid may be grasped with blunt-tipped forceps (**Fig. 14**) and elevated to facilitate examination of its bulbar surface.

Raised or ulcerated lesions along the free margin and palpebral surface of the third eyelid and at the temporal limbus should be considered as strongly suspect for squamous cell carcinoma (**Fig. 15**). Infectious agents such as *Moraxella bovis, Mycoplasma* spp, and *Chlamydophila* spp are frequent causes of conjunctivitis in ruminants.[34-36] After application of a topical anesthetic (proparacaine ophthalmic solution), conjunctival swabs may be obtained for cytologic examination, culture, or polymerase chain reaction (PCR) assays to facilitate identification of the underlying etiologic agent. One should consult with the diagnostic laboratory performing the testing beforehand to determine their preferred transport media and sample handling, especially in regard of *Mycoplasma* and *Chlamydophila*.

Cornea

The surface of the cornea should be examined with focused illumination, ideally using a Finnoff transilluminator and source of magnification such as a head loupe (**Fig. 16**). Normal cornea is smooth, transparent, and glossy with a reflective surface. Blood vessels should not be present within the cornea. Fine, branching vessels that originate from the conjunctiva signify surface ocular disease (ie, chronic irritation or ulceration). Short, straight, deep vessels that originate at the limbus signify a deep keratitis or intraocular disease (anterior uveitis or glaucoma). White to pink to red, raised lesions of the corneal surface may signify granulation tissue and normal corneal healing after trauma or a deep corneal ulceration. However if the lesion is ulcerated, associated with the temporal limbus, and particularly if the adjacent conjunctiva is involved, one should be highly suspicious of squamous cell carcinoma.

The cornea should be free of opacities. White opacities may signify the presence of lipid, calcium, or fibrosis within the corneal stroma. A beige or milky appearance to the cornea often signifies the presence of inflammatory cells within the corneal stroma, particularly if noted in association with corneal ulceration (**Fig. 17**). A bluish-gray, "steamy" appearance, either in focal regions or generalized, typically signifies corneal edema. Corneal malacia causes the affected portion of the cornea to assume a gelatinous appearance as proteinases and collagenases break down the normal collagen structure of the corneal stroma. Immediate, aggressive therapeutic intervention is recommended to prevent corneal rupture. The presence of a brown to black protrusion, which may or may not be covered with a yellow to ochre layer (fibrin), should be considered highly suspicious for a corneal rupture and iris prolapse. Further evaluation of the anterior chamber depth and position of the pupil are critical. Tan to brown flecks or consolidations along the corneal endothelium are keratic precipitates and are accumulations of inflammatory cells. Keratic precipitates tend to occur along the ventromedial aspect of the cornea and may therefore be obscured by the third eyelid,

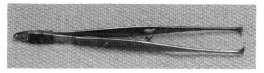

Fig. 14. Graephe fixation forceps, useful for elevation of the third eyelid.

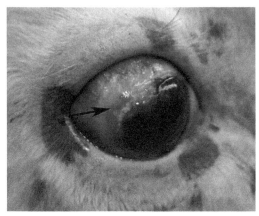

Fig. 15. Conjunctival squamous cell carcinoma (*arrow*) in a 10-year-old Hereford bull. Note the raised, ulcerated appearance of the lesion.

particularly if it is elevated. Keratic precipitates indicate the presence of anterior uveitis.

Instillation of fluorescein dye aids in the identification of corneal ulceration. Moisten the tip of the fluorescein dye strip with saline or eyewash and apply a drop to the dorsal bulbar conjunctiva. Alternatively, place the tip of the fluorescein strip in a tuberculin syringe containing 0.5 mL of saline or eyewash. Break the tip off from a 25-gauge needle and attach the needle hub to the syringe. Spray the fluorescein into the eye, being careful not to contact the globe with the hub of the needle. Normal cornea should not take up fluorescein dye. Areas of fluorescein retention signify breaks in the corneal epithelium. If the cornea retains its normal contour in the area of fluorescein uptake, then the lesion is likely superficial. If the corneal contour is altered in the area of fluorescein uptake, particularly if the area has a crater-form appearance, then the ulceration involves the corneal stroma and is likely septic. Corneal swabs for cytologic evaluation and bacterial culture and sensitivity are highly recommended, as is an aggressive therapeutic regimen.

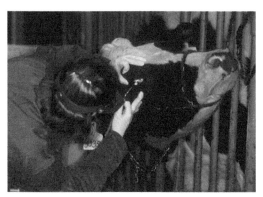

Fig. 16. Examining the anterior segment of a cow using a Finnoff transilluminator and magnifying head loupe.

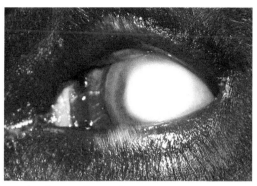

Fig. 17. Angus heifer with infectious bovine keratoconjunctivitis. Note the presence of deep and superficial corneal vascularization as well as a dense area of cellular infiltrate centrally.

Anterior Chamber

The normal anterior chamber is filled with clear aqueous humor. The presence of blood (hyphema), fibrin, increased protein (flare), or inflammatory cells (hypopyon) is abnormal (**Fig. 18**). Aqueous flare is best detected by directing a slit-beam of light or the smallest spot size of light from a direct ophthalmoscope across the anterior chamber. Do not look through the viewing aperture, but instead from a 45° angle. If one can see the light as it traverses the aqueous humor, much like one can visualize light from a movie projector (the Tyndall effect), then aqueous flare is present. Flare signifies an increase in the protein content of the aqueous humor and is the hallmark of anterior uveitis. As uveitis in ruminants is often associated with systemic disease (eg, neonatal septicemia; bacterial septicemia associated with severe mastitis, metritis, or traumatic reticuloperitonitis; leptospirosis; listeriosis; and EHV-1 in camelids), one should perform a complete physical examination.[37–39]

One should also note changes in the depth of the anterior chamber. A shallowing of the anterior chamber occurs with corneal or globe perforation causing a loss of aqueous humor, mass lesions within the anterior chamber, iris "bombe" (the anterior bulging of the iris that occurs after 360° posterior synechia), and anterior subluxation of the lens (the lens remains behind the iridal face, but has displaced anteriorly). An

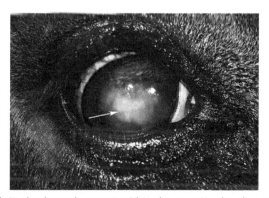

Fig. 18. Central fibrin clot (*arrow*) present within the anterior chamber of a mini Zebu bull presenting for uveitis and diarrhea.

increased anterior chamber depth occurs with keratoconus (anterior projection of the cornea), anterior lens luxation (lens is noted within the anterior chamber and displaces the iris posteriorly), and posterior lens luxation (lens is noted within the posterior segment).

Iris and Pupillary Margin

The contour and coloration of the iridal surface should be evaluated. The iris may be brown or blue in color, or a combination of brown and blue (heterochromia iridis). The corpora nigra (or pupillary rough in camelids) should be evaluated for the presence of cystic structures (uveal cysts) or adhesions to either the lens (posterior synechia) or cornea (anterior synechia). Any strands or adhesions should be inspected to determine if they represent synechia (adhesions after previous inflammation or trauma) or persistent pupillary membranes (congenital lesions). Persistent pupillary membranes typically arise from the iris collarette, which is located halfway between the pupillary margin and the base of the iris. Synechia may occur at any location, but most often are present along the pupillary margin or along the base of the iris (peripheral anterior synechia). Mass lesions can be transilluminated to differentiate melanomas (solid) from iris cysts (allow light to pass). The surface of the iris should be inspected for the presence of neovascularization, which can develop from chronic uveitis or long-standing retinal detachment. The pupillary margin should be ovoid in shape, centrally located, and freely movable. Abnormal pupil shaped is termed dyscoria. Incorrect pupil location is termed corectopia and occurs as a congenital lesion. Lack of normal mobility may occur because of posterior synechia, mass lesions within the iris, cellular infiltrates within the iris, or iris atrophy (pupil is dilated and constricts poorly due to loss of sphincter muscle tone). If not previously assessed, pupillary light reflexes should be evaluated.

Lens

The pupil should be pharmacologically dilated with 1% tropicamide ophthalmic solution to allow complete visualization of the lens and posterior segment. Mydriasis occurs within 20 to 30 minutes after application. The lens should lie behind the iris within the patellar fossa. Dislocation or luxation of the lens may occur after damage to the zonular fibers through either trauma or chronic intraocular inflammation. No portion of the lens equator is visible when the lens is positioned normally. The lens should be completely clear with a smooth convex anterior surface and concave posterior surface. Direct illumination and retroillumination facilitate detection of opacities (cataracts), which will appear white with direct illumination and dark when retroilluminated (**Fig. 19**). The cataracts may be categorized by location (anterior, posterior, equatorial, nuclear, cortical, capsular) and extent of lenticular involvement (incipient, immature, mature, and hypermature). Cataracts may occur as congenital lesions (BVD exposure in utero between days 76 and 150 of gestation in cattle[40]) or develop secondary to trauma and inflammation. Small opacities do not typically impair vision and may therefore be missed during examination, particularly if the pupil is not dilated.

Vitreous

The normal vitreous is a transparent, gel-like structure filling the posterior segment. The presence of blood or vasculature within the posterior segment is abnormal and may signify persistence of the hyaloid artery. In young ruminants, a nonpatent remnant of the hyaloid artery is often noted arising from the center of the optic disk and is termed Bergmeister's papilla (**Fig. 20**). Inflammation within the ciliary body may cause an accumulation of inflammatory cells within the anterior vitreous. Small, refractile

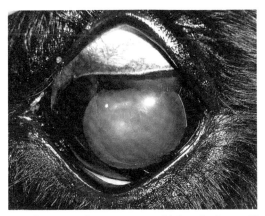

Fig. 19. Posterior cortical cataract in an 11-year-old female llama. The cataract did not appear to impair her vision and had not been noted previously.

spheres composed of calcium and phospholipids signify asteroid hyalosis, which rarely has any impact on vision.

Fundus

The retina and optic disk are best evaluated using a transilluminator and 15- to 20-diopter indirect lens, or a direct ophthalmoscope focused at 0 to −4 diopters. To perform indirect ophthalmoscopy, the transilluminator is rested against the cheek and held in the dominant hand. Working at arm's length from the animal's eye, obtain a strong tapetal reflex. Then move the lens, held by the thumb and index finger, into position in front of the eye. Pull the lens slowly back toward yourself until the fundic image completely fills the lens (**Fig. 21**).

The normal bovine retina has 3 to 4 major venules accompanied by arterioles. The superior venule and arteriole may twist about each other. The vessels merge on the surface of the optic disk, which is shaped as a horizontally flattened oval and is white, pink, gray, orange, or tan in color. The tapetal fundus is yellow to bluish purple and is uniformly stippled by end-on capillaries (stars of Winslow). The nontapetal fundus is generally a uniform shade of brown. The normal ovine fundus is similar to that of cattle

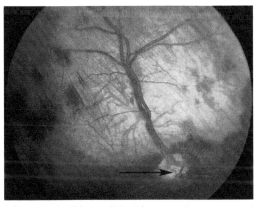

Fig. 20. The fundus of a 1-week-old camelid with a prominent Bergmeister papilla (*arrow*).

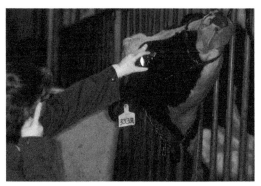

Fig. 21. Proper technique to perform indirect ophthalmoscopy. Note the position of the examiner, transilluminator, and the lens with regard to the cow's eye.

(**Fig. 22**). The superior venule and arteriole are less apt to twine about one another. The tapetal fundus is more often greenish blue. The optic disk has a kidney shape. Goats have more retinal blood vessels with 5 to 8 venules often present. The optic disk is often rounded with a surrounding pigment disk. The camelid fundus lacks a tapetum. The retinal vascular pattern is similar to that of cattle. The amount of pigmentation varies according to coat color. The optic disk is slightly ovoid in shape (**Fig. 23**). All ruminants may have a small fibrous projection extending from the physiologic pit of the optic nerve into the vitreous, which is a remnant of the hyaloid artery and is called Bergmeister's papilla.

One should first closely examine the optic nerve for its size (small = atrophy or optic nerve aplasia/hypoplasia; enlarged = excessive myelination, a variation of normal, or papilledema due to compression of the nerve fibers, or optic neuritis), color (pale = atrophy; hyperemic = neuritis), and overlying vasculature (thin caliber = retinal degeneration or severe anemia; engorged = vasculitis ± optic neuritis). Then examine the tapetal fundus for variations in reflectivity. Areas of increased reflectivity signify areas of retinal thinning. Areas of decreased reflectivity signify areas with an inflammatory or cellular infiltrate within the retina or the subretinal space. The pigmented portion of the fundus should be examined for areas of increased pigment deposition (black clumps of pigment), areas of gray to pink coloration caused by cellular infiltrates within the

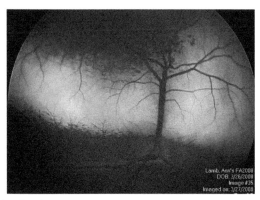

Fig. 22. Normal ovine fundus.

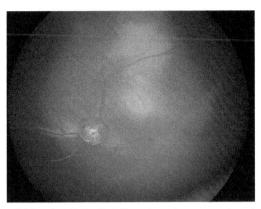

Fig. 23. Normal camelid fundus. Note that they do not possess a tapetum lucidum.

retina or subretinal space, or areas with loss of pigmentation due to retinal degeneration or atrophy. Colobomas of the choroid are relatively common in cattle, especially Herefords, and appear as white to gray outpouchings within the fundus that appear to lack a normal overlying retina. Colobomas may involve the optic nerve or the retina, and vary in size. The effect on vision depends on the size and location.

THERAPEUTIC REGIMENS

The therapeutic regimen selected must be tailored based on the number of animals affected, their intended or current usage, and the feasibility of applying topical medications versus parenteral administration. When dealing with animals used for meat or milk production, one must always be cognizant of the recommended WDI to avoid medication residues. WDIs listed in this article were current at the time of publication and are those required within the United States. An excellent resource to obtain updated information regarding WDI is the Food Animal Residue Avoidance and Depletion Program (FARAD) home page, located at www.farad.org. As little systemic absorption occurs after application of the diagnostic medications mentioned earlier in this article (fluorescein stain, tropicamide ophthalmic solution, proparacaine ophthalmic solution), a withdrawal time of 1 day after administration for meat and milk should be sufficient (M. Gatz Riddell, DVM, personal communication, 2009).

Keratoconjunctivitis

In cattle, most cases of keratoconjunctivitis result from *Moraxella bovis*. Drugs labeled for treatment of infectious bovine keratoconjunctivitis in the United States are long-acting tetracycline (11 mg/kg intramuscular [IM] or subcutaneous [SQ] with 2 injections 48 to 72 hours apart, WDI of 96 hours milk and 28 days meat) and tulathromycin (Draxxin) (2.5 mg/kg SQ in the neck region once, not for use in female dairy cattle older than 20 months, 18 days meat WDI). Other therapeutic options constitute extralabel drug use. One option is bulbar subconjunctival injection of 300,000 IU of procaine penicillin G (**Fig. 24**) (suggested 22–36 hours milk WDI and 12 days meat WDI[41]), although clinical trials have not supported its efficacy.[42] Other options that have proven more effective include systemic administration of florfenicol (NuFlor) (20 mg/kg IM for 2 injections 24 hours apart or 40 mg/kg SQ as a single dose, not for use in female dairy cattle older than 20 months, 28 days meat WDI after IM injection and 38 days meat WDI after SQ injection) and ceftiofur (Excede) (6.6 mg/kg SQ at the

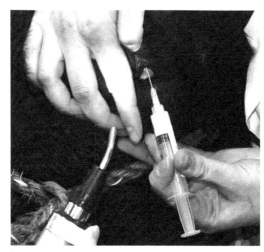

Fig. 24. Injection of procaine penicillin G under the bulbar conjunctiva.

base of the ear once, no milk WDI and 13 days meat WDI).[43,44] None of these antimicrobials are approved for use in calves intended for veal. In severely affected eyes, placement of a temporary tarsorrhaphy or third eyelid flap may provide additional protection from the environment and prevent exposure in globes with a markedly distended cornea.

Sheep, goats, and camelids may be treated with topical tetracycline or tetracycline—polymyxin b ophthalmic ointment 3 to 4 times daily in small herds or flocks for which this is practical. Tetracycline is selected for use because it is effective against both *Chlamydophila* and *Mycoplasma*. Alternatively one may administer tetracycline parenterally. After administration of a single dose of injectable oxytetracycline (6.6–11.0 mg/kg [3–5 mg/lb]), FARAD recommends a discard period of at least 96 hours and then testing milk for antibiotic residues.[45] Following multiple doses or high doses, a milk discard time of 144 hours should be observed, followed by residue testing.[45] The meat WDI is 5 days.[46] After topical administration of tetracyclines or tetracycline with polymyxin b, there is no required withdrawal time.[46]

Uveitis

The therapeutic goals when treating uveitis are suppressing inflammation, dilating the pupil, alleviating pain, and treating the underlying cause. To suppress inflammation one should administer either corticosteroids or nonsteroidal anti-inflammatory drugs (NSAIDs). Topically one may administer neomycin polymyxin b dexamethasone ophthalmic solution or ointment at a frequency of every 2 to every 24 hours, depending on the severity of the inflammation. One can also use dexamethasone 0.1% ophthalmic solution topically at the same frequency. Dexamethasone, neomycin, and polymyxin are all approved for systemic usage in food animal species. No WDI is required when these products are applied topically to the eye (US FARAD, personal communication, 2009). However, products containing neomycin may not be used in veal calves.

One may also inject dexamethasone sodium phosphate (0.5–1 mg) under the bulbar conjunctiva (the portion overlying the sclera) to increase drug concentrations and limit the frequency at which medications must be applied. Again the WDI is zero days, as dexamethasone is approved for systemic usage in food animal species with a zero WDI. In camelids one may also use topical 1% prednisolone acetate ophthalmic solution or topical NSAIDs such as flurbiprofen 0.03% ophthalmic solution.

If the inflammation involves the vitreous or retina, then medications must be administered systemically to achieve therapeutic levels within the posterior segment. Dexamethasone is approved for usage in food animals and has no WDI. However, its use in the last trimester of pregnancy is contraindicated, as it may induce parturition. If one wishes to use a systemic NSAID, flunixin meglumine is the only NSAID in the United States labeled for use in beef and dairy cattle.[47] It is approved for intravenous administration only at 1.1 to 2.2 mg/kg with a WDI of 4 days for meat and 36 hours for milk. Intramuscular and subcutaneous injections cause significant tissue damage and prolonged drug clearance, and are considered illegal based on conditions set forth by the Animal Medicinal Drug Use Clarification Act (AMDUCA).[47] Although aspirin is commonly used in food animals, FARAD strongly discourages its usage due to its questionable legality and the availability of flunixin meglumine as an approved alternative.[47]

In addition to suppression of inflammation using NSAIDs or corticosteroids, dilation of the pupil is an important component of treatment for uveitis. Mydriasis is crucial, as it alleviates the pain from uveitis, much of which occurs due to spasm of the ciliary muscle. Mydriasis also limits the formation of posterior synechia, thereby minimizing visual obstruction. Topical atropine 1% ophthalmic solution or ointment is applied 2 to 8 times daily until the pupil dilates, and continued every 24 to 48 hours to maintain the dilation.[48] Administration of atropine also assists in stabilization of the blood aqueous barrier. As there is some systemic absorption of atropine after topical administration, a withdrawal time of at least 1 day would be recommended (M. Gatz Riddell, DVM, personal communication, 2009). Subconjunctival administration of 2 mg atropine can also be performed to facilitate treatment.[49] At this dosage, a meat WDI of 7 days and milk WDI of 24 hours should be sufficient.[3]

The final component in uveitis therapy is treatment of the underlying cause. Multiple conditions such as leptospirosis, traumatic reticuloperitonitis, mastitis, and neonatal septicemia can result in uveitis. A complete physical examination is indicated to ensure detection of these conditions. Discussion of their management is beyond the scope of this article. The reader is directed to the many excellent large animal internal medicine textbooks for a detailed discussion of therapeutic options.

SUMMARY

A complete ocular examination is critical when presented with patients suffering from an ocular complaint. An ocular examination can also provide additional information when confronted with a systemic disease for which the cause is not easily ascertained. Utilizing the step-wise approach and diagnostic equipment outlined in this article, the examination can be easily completed on the farm. The therapeutic regimens discussed address the key components of therapy for both keratoconjunctivitis and uveitis; the two conditions most commonly encountered in food animal practice.

REFERENCES

1. Knight AP. Xylazine. Journal of the American Veterinary Medical Association 1980;176(5):454–5.
2. Taylor P. Anesthesia in sheep and goats. In: Melling M, Alder M, editors. Sheep and goat practice 2. London: WB Saunders; 1998. p. 104–11.

3. Craigmill AL, Rangel-Lugo M, Damian P, et al. Extralabel use of tranquilizers and general anesthetics. J Am Vet Med Assoc 1997;211(3):302–4.

4. Cullen CL, Webb AA. Ocular manifestations of systemic diseases. In: Gelatt K, editor. Part 4: food animals. 4th edition. Veterinary ophthalmology, vol. 2. 4th edition. Ames (IA): Blackwell; 2007. p. 1617–43.

5. Samuelson D. Ophthalmic anatomy. In: Gelatt K, editor. Veterinary ophthalmology, vol. 1. Ames (IA): Blackwell Publishing; 2007. p. 63.

6. Prince J, Diesem C, Eglitis I, et al. Anatomy and histology of the eye and orbit in domestic animals. Springfield (IL): CC Thomas; 1960.

7. Neathery MW, Miller WJ. Metabolism and toxicity of cadmium, mercury, and lead in animals: a review. J Dairy Sci 1975;58(12):1767–81.

8. McGuirk SM. Polioencephalomalacia. Vet Clin North Am Food Anim Pract 1987; 3(1):107–17.

9. Gould DH. Polioencephalomalacia. J Anim Sci 1998;76(1):309–14.

10. MacDonald DW, Christian RG, Chalmers GA. Infectious thromboembolic meningoencephalitis: literature review and occurrence in Alberta, 1969–71. Can Vet J 1973;14(3):57–61.

11. Lindberg A, Stokstad M, Loken T, et al. Indirect transmission of bovine viral diarrhoea virus at calving and during the postparturient period. Vet Rec 2004; 154(15):463–7.

12. Stokstad M, Loken T. Pestivirus in cattle: experimentally induced persistent infection in calves. J Vet Med B Infect Dis Vet Public Health 2002;49(10):494–501.

13. Binns W, Shupe JL, Keeler RF, et al. Chronologic evaluation of teratogenicity in sheep fed *Veratrum californicum*. J Am Vet Med Assoc 1965;147(8):839–42.

14. Rebhun WC. Diseases of the bovine orbit and globe. J Am Vet Med Assoc 1979; 175(2):171–5.

15. Ward JL, Rebhun WC. Chronic frontal sinusitis in dairy cattle: 12 cases (1978–1989). J Am Vet Med Assoc 1992;201(2):326–8.

16. McConnon JM, White ME, Smith MC, et al. Pendular nystagmus in dairy cattle. J Am Vet Med Assoc 1983;182(8):812–3.

17. Braun U, Stehle C, Ehrensperger F. Clinical findings and treatment of listeriosis in 67 sheep and goats. Vet Rec 2002;150(2):38–42.

18. Brenner J, Perl S, Lahav D, et al. An unusual outbreak of malignant catarrhal fever in a beef herd in Israel. J Vet Med B Infect Dis Vet Public Health 2002;49(6):304–7.

19. Gionfriddo JP. Ophthalmology of South American camelids: llamas, alpacas, guanacos, and vicunas. In: Howard JL, Smith RA, editors. Current veterinary therapy 4: food animal practice. 4th edition. Philadelphia: W.B. Saunders; 1999. p. 644–8.

20. Wyman M. Eye diseases of sheep and goats. Vet Clin North Am Large Anim Pract 1983;5(3):657–75.

21. McManus TJ. Report of entropion in newborn lambs. Aust Vet J 1960;36:91–2.

22. Crowley JP, McGloughlin P. Hereditary entropion in lambs. Vet Rec 1963;75: 1104–6.

23. Green LE, Berriatua E, Morgan KL. The prevalence and risk factors for congenital entropion in intensively reared lambs in south west England. Prev Vet Med 1995; 24(1):15–21.

24. Evans A. Diseases of the skin: bacterial diseases. In: Smith B, editor. Large animal internal medicine. St Louis (MO): Mosby; 1990. p. 1267.

25. Smith B. Large animal internal medicine. St Louis (MO): Mosby; 1990.

26. Stannard A. Diseases of the skin: mycotic diseases. In: Smith B, editor. Large animal internal medicine. St Louis (MO): Mosby; 1990. p. 1272–3.

27. Moore CP, Whitley RD. Ophthalmic diseases of small domestic ruminants. Vet Clin North Am Large Anim Pract 1984;6(3):641–65.

28. Blood D, Radostits O. Veterinary medicine. 7th edition. London: Bailliere Tindall; 1989.

29. Kako MD, al-Sultan II, Saleem AN. Studies of sheep experimentally poisoned with *Hypericum perforatum*. Vet Hum Toxicol 1993;35(4):298–300.

30. Smith MC. Caprine dermatologic problems: a review. J Am Vet Med Assoc 1981; 178(7):724–9.

31. Moore CP. Diseases of the eye. In: Smith B, editor. Large animal internal medicine. St Louis (MO): Mosby; 1990. p. 1197–203.

32. Gionfriddo JR. Update on llama medicine. Ophthalmology. Vet Clin North Am Food Anim Pract 1994;10(2):371–82.

33. Kennedy MJ, Moraiko DT, Goonewardene L. A study on the prevalence and intensity of occurrence of *Thelazia skrjabini* (Nematoda: Thelazioidea) in cattle in central Alberta, Canada. J Parasitol 1990;76(2):196–200.

34. Storz J. Overview of animal diseases induced by chlamydial infections. Boca Raton (FL): CRC Press Inc; 1988.

35. Rosenbusch RF, Knudtson WU. Bovine mycoplasmal conjunctivitis: experimental reproduction and characterization of the disease. Cornell Vet 1980; 70(4):307–20.

36. Slatter DH, Edwards ME, Hawkins CD, et al. A national survey of the clinical features, treatment and importance of infectious bovine keratoconjunctivitis. Aust Vet J 1982;59(3):69–72.

37. Rebhun WC. Ocular manifestations of systemic diseases in cattle. Vet Clin North Am Large Anim Pract 1984;6(3):623–39.

38. Rebhun WC, Jenkins DH, Riis RC, et al. An epizootic of blindness and encephalitis associated with a herpesvirus indistinguishable from equine herpesvirus I in a herd of alpacas and llamas. J Am Vet Med Assoc 1988;192(7):953–6.

39. Mee JE, Rea M. Baled silage-associated uveitis in cows. Vet Rec 1989;125(1):25.

40. Bistner SI, Rubin LF, Saunders LZ. The ocular lesions of bovine viral diarrhea—mucosal disease. Pathol Vet 1970;7:272–86.

41. Payne MA, Craigmill A, Riviere JE, et al. Extralabel use of penicillin in food animals. J Am Vet Med Assoc 2006;229(9):1401–3.

42. Allen LJ, George LW, Willits NH. Effect of penicillin or penicillin and dexamethasone in cattle with infectious bovine keratoconjunctivitis. J Am Vet Med Assoc 1995;206(8):1200–3.

43. Angelos JA, Dueger EI, George LW, et al. Efficacy of florfenicol for treatment of naturally occurring infectious bovine keratoconjunctivitis. Journal of the American Veterinary Medical Association 2000;216(1):62–4.

44. Dueger EL, George LW, Angelos JA, et al. Efficacy of a long-acting formulation of ceftiofur crystalline-free acid for the treatment of naturally occurring infectious bovine keratoconjunctivitis. Am J Vet Res 2004;65(9):1185–8.

45. Martin-Jimenez T, Craigmill AL, Riviere JE. Extralabel use of oxytetracycline. J Am Vet Med Assoc 1997;211(1):42–4.

46. Webb AI, Baynes RE, Craigmill AL, et al. Drugs approved for small ruminants. J Am Vet Med Assoc 2004;224(4):520–3.

47. Smith G, Davis J, Tell L, et al. Extralabel use of nonsteroidal anti-inflammatory drugs in cattle. Journal of the American Veterinary Medical Association 2008; 232(5):697–701.

48. Klauss G, Constantinescu GM. Nonhypotensive autonomic agents in veterinary ophthalmology. Vet Clin North Am Small Anim Pract 2004;34(3):777–800.

49. Ward DA. Clinical pharmacology and therapeutics: part 3. In: Gelatt K, editor. Veterinary ophthalmology. 3rd edition. Baltimore (MD): Lippincott, Williams, and Wilkins; 1999. p. 336–7.
50. Reibold T, Geiser D, Goble D. Large animal anesthesia: principles and techniques. 2nd edition. Ames (IA): Iowa State Press; 1995.
51. Riviere J, Papich M. Veterinary pharmacology and therapeutics. 9th edition. Ames (IA): Wiley-Blackwell; 2009.
52. Fowler M. Medicine and surgery of South American camelids. 2nd edition. Ames (IA): Iowa State University Press; 1998.

Surgical Treatment of the Eye in Farm Animals

Rachel Shaw-Edwards, BA, VetMB, MRCVS

KEYWORDS

- Eye surgery • Ocular surgery • Farm animals
- Surgical treatment

Although many eye conditions can be managed medically, several require surgical intervention. This article aims to review those conditions with surgical treatment options before going on to consider the various aspects of surgery itself, whether that be in the field or in a hospital setting. Often the surgery one would ideally like to perform is limited by geographic issues of transporting the animal to a surgical facility, and thus attempts have to be made to undertake the best operative procedures one can, given the field conditions available. Even more so, economic factors often limit the type of operations one would wish to carry out. Here, rather than reduce the surgical techniques discussed to the lowest common denominator, the author seeks to explore what is possible in the best situations, trusting that the reader can modify the operations described to fit the environment and animal they are faced with.

CONDITIONS POTENTIALLY REQUIRING SURGICAL INTERVENTIONS
The Orbit and Globe

Proptosis, protrusion of the eye from the orbit, is commonly caused by trauma. But, whatever the reason for this protrusion, the eye is exposed and requires frequent cleansing and moistening until further action can be taken. If the eye has ruptured or there is a significant risk of a blind, painful globe remaining, then an enucleation will be required (**Box 1**).

Orbital inflammation or cellulitis can be managed medically with hot packs, broad spectrum antibiotics, and antiinflammatory drugs. In some cases, however, the inflammation persists despite treatment; usually the swelling will localize and a fluid pocket can be detected by palpation or ultrasound. Once detected, the area should be aseptically prepared and aspirated to allow ventral drainage.

Lymphosarcoma is the most common orbital tumor in cattle[1]; it causes subacute or chronic onset exophthalmos. Digital palpation of the retrobulbar area, cytologic sampling, or biopsy should be performed to differentiate this from excessive or prolapsed orbital fat. The prognosis for survival in animals showing clinical signs is poor, especially those with bilateral exophthalmos.[2] However, for a cow in late

Department of Veterinary Medicine, University of Cambridge, Madingley Road, Cambridge CB3 0ES, UK
E-mail address: edwards.vet@gmail.com

Vet Clin Food Anim 26 (2010) 459–476
doi:10.1016/j.cvfa.2010.09.007
0749-0720/10/$ – see front matter © 2010 Elsevier Inc. All rights reserved.

Box 1
Removing the eye

Enucleation

1. Suture/clamp the upper and lower eyelids together (ford interlocking pattern).

2. Make a circumferential skin incision approximately 1 cm from the eyelid edges.

3. Transect the medial and lateral canthal ligaments and each of the rectus muscles at the point of insertion.

4. Dissect around the globe.

5. Clamp and transect retrobulbar muscle and optic nerve sheath.

6. Close skin incision using nonabsorbable suture material. The pattern used is the surgeon's choice, a trampoline suture will provide a better final cosmetic appearance and placing interrupted sutures in the medial portion will allow drainage, but could also allow infection to enter.

7. To aid hemostasis, apply a pressure bandage for 24 hours.

Exenteration

1. Suture the lower eyelids and incise the skin as described for enucleation.

2. Dissect everything away from the bony orbit, rectus muscles included.

3. Transect the optic nerve and retrobulbar muscle as close to the bony orbit as possible.

4. Close the skin as previously described. In these cases, a drain may be necessary despite the risk of infection.

Evisceration and placement of intrascleral prosthesis

1. Perform general anesthesia.

2. Prepare the surgical area, including a nasolacrimal lavage.

3. Retract the eyelids, either by speculum or stay sutures.

4. Incise the conjunctiva dorsally at the 12-o'clock position approximately 1 cm from the limbus depending on the size of your patient.

5. Extend the incision parallel to the limbus from 12 o'clock to 2 o'clock and 10 o'clock.

6. Use a blade to make a sharp incision through the sclera at 12 o'clock.

7. Suction out any aqueous and vitreous fluid that remains. Always point the suction device caudally, that is, away from the cornea.

8. Extend the scleral incision to 10 o'clock and 2 o'clock using thermocautery.

9. Separate the choroid from the sclera using a small spatula. Once dissected free, remove the choroid using 2 tissue forceps. If any choroid is left attached to the sclera it will continue to bleed and must be removed.

10. Select the implant. Available implants should range from 2-mm less to 2-mm greater in diameter than the diameter of the normal eye.

11. Insert the implant. A total of 4 to 6 stay sutures placed in the wound margin allow the sclera to be elevated up and over the ball as it is pushed into place.

12. Close the incision. The sclera should be closed with absorbable sutures in a simple interrupted pattern and then over sewn with a simple continuous pattern. The conjunctiva can be closed with a simple continuous pattern.

13. A temporary tarsorrhaphy should be performed to protect the surgical site.

gestation it may be long enough to allow her to give birth to her calf. During this period, palliative treatment is essential to protect the eye, thus minimizing the pain and damage caused by exposure. What form this treatment takes will depend on the severity of exophthalmos. Mild cases may only require the application of a topical artificial tear preparation; whereas, with increasing severity permanent and complete tarsorrhaphy, enucleation, or exenteration[3] may be warranted (see **Box 1**; **Fig. 1**). Where cost is not prohibitive and visual appearance is important, evisceration followed by placement of a prosthesis may be considered.

Although prolapse of the retrobulbar fat pad is uncommon, it can greatly alter the appearance of the eye and may compromise visual function. To resolve both of these issues the fat pad can be removed surgically and this procedure is described later (**Box 2**).

Head Trauma

Traumatic injuries to the head are common in ruminants, and serious ones should always be treated as an emergency. The animal should be restrained to avoid any further damage occurring. Corneal lacerations, corneoscleral avulsions, and scleral ruptures should be surgically repaired as soon as possible. Even if the cornea appears normal at the time, it should be closely monitored for several days because the epithelium can slough.

Fractures of the orbit are less common in ruminants than in the equine; the frontal, and zygomatic bones are more commonly fractured in these species. Diagnosis of such abnormalities is usually easily done by palpation if there is a history of trauma, but skull radiographs, when possible, are a valuable aid allowing the extent of the damage to be properly evaluated. Eye motility should also be evaluated; forced ductions of the globe may be required to do this. Those fractures with normal ocular motility and without fracture fragment displacement can be managed with symptomatic treatment: cold compresses, antiinflammatory drugs, and analgesia. Cases with sinus compromise, displaced fragments, marked facial deformity, or displacement of the globe require fracture repair. This procedure is easiest in the first 24 to 48 hours assuming the patients are in a suitable condition for general anesthesia. If eyelid function has been compromised, then eye lubricants must be used frequently to prevent desiccation of the cornea. The globe can be protected with a membrana nictitans flap (**Box 3**) or tarsorrhaphy (**Box 4**).

The Eyelid

Entropion, in turning of the eyelid, is a common condition seen especially in lambs (**Fig. 2**). In newborns it can be anatomic and may have a genetic component to it,[4] or alternatively associated with dehydration or microphthalmos. In other age groups it may be secondary to squinting caused by eye pain or eyelid scarring. Whatever the cause, in turning results in eyelid hair touching the cornea, described as trichiasis; this is irritating and painful and surgical intervention is required (**Box 5**). Treatment is often by injection of a long-acting antibiotic bleb into the palpebral skin to affect out-turning (**Fig. 3**) or even injection of air in the same area for a short-lasting effect. More severe in turning, as seen in **Fig. 4**, requires surgery with the Hotz-Celsus technique, removing a significant area of eyelid skin to achieve sufficient out turning. Ectropion, rolling out of the eyelid, does not usually require treatment unless there is concurrent ocular disease that may be attributable to the deformation (**Fig. 5**).

Eyelid lacerations that involve the eyelid margin must be repaired surgically as soon as possible (**Box 6**), preserving as much of the original tissue as possible. The eyelid margin is essential for correct eyelid function to maintain ocular health, through

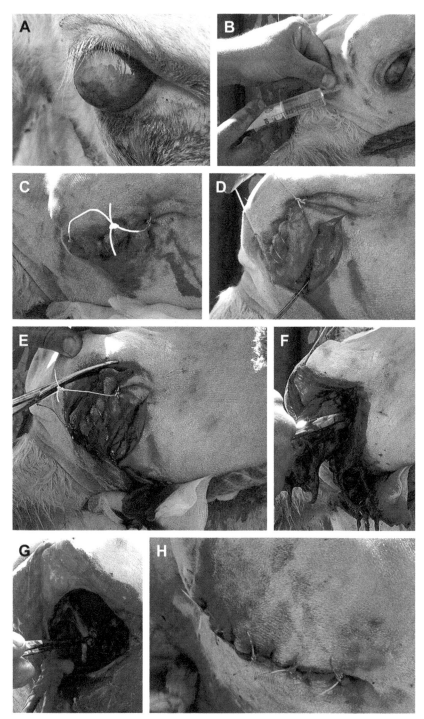

Fig. 1. (*A*) Blind painful eye requiring enucleation. (*B*) Injection for Petersen block. (*C*) Tarsoraphy prior to enucleation. (*D*) Initial palpebral incision. (*E*) Second palpebral incision. (*F*) Commencing globe removal. (*G*) Globe removal complete. (*H*) Suture placement closing socket.

spreading of the tear film and protection from exposure. Loss or unsuitable repair can result is chronic discomfort caused by exposure keratitis, irritation from hairs, and keratoconjunctivitis.

Conjunctival flaps can be used but result in a more opaque scar; nictitating membrane flaps and temporary tarsorrhaphies should not be used because they cause corneal irritation and can result in increased intraocular pressure.

Box 2
Removing a mass

Excision

Excision of a mass in the eyelid creates a surgical dilemma. On the one hand, the mass needs to be removed, and in the case of neoplastic mass, the need for complete removal and clean margins is important. However, from a functional point of view, every piece of eyelid tissue is important and, thus, when removing part of the eyelid it is vital that we try to remove as little as possible, especially of the margin. With this in mind, the older techniques of wedge excision have been superseded by the so-called tent excisions, and it is the latter that is subsequently described.

1. Prepare and clean the surgical and surrounding area.

2. Examine the eyelid to determine the extent of the mass.

3. Clamp around the lesion to aid hemostasis. This procedure is best done with lid forceps or clamps with a solid lower plate.

4. Use a scalpel blade to make 2 incisions: one on either side of the mass and both perpendicular to the eyelid margin.

5. Make 2 more incisions in a *V* shape caudal to the mass, joining the edge of the previous incisions together at a point.

6. Remove the portion of eyelid with the mass.

7. Close the incision in 3 layers using absorbable sutures in a figure-of-eight pattern. The deep layer must contain the tarsal plate and contain the orbicularis oculi muscle. The middle layer should be the subcuticular tissues. The final layer is the skin and this can be closed routinely. The first suture is the most important and must result in perfect alignment and apposition of the wound and eyelid margin. A stent may be used to aid support of the lid.

H-blepharoplasty

1. Make 2 full-thickness skin incisions: one on each side of the mass and both perpendicular to the eyelid margin.

2. Make 1 full-thickness skin incision to create an *H*, which is at the caudal border of the mass, parallel to the eye-lid margin connecting the previous 2 incisions.

3. Remove a triangle of skin from either exterior side of the *H*. The 3 corners of the triangle are the point at which the cross bar meets the perpendicular incisions, the top of the perpendicular incision (that is, the end that does not meet the eyelid margin), and a point halfway between these 2 points exterior to the *H* at such a distance as to form an equilateral triangle with the other 2 points.

4. Excise the mass by dissection from the underlying tissues.

5. Dissect the remaining part of the *H*; that is, the half not in contact with the eyelid margin, away from its subcutaneous tissues, this will form the skin graft.

6. Slide the skin graft until the margin is aligned with the eyelid margin

7. Suture the graft using non-absorbable suture material and an interrupted suture pattern

Membrana nictitans excision

1. Administer preoperative topical antibiotics for 24 hours before the procedure.
2. Sedate patient.
3. Administer topical and local anesthesia.
4. Lavage the conjunctival sac.
5. Retropulse (to drive/push back) the globe.
6. Grab the free margin of the third eyelid with hemostats and evert.
7. If removing a tumor, check that there is enough normal tissue present to allow complete removal.
8. Stretch the membrane as far laterally as possible.
9. Clamp Kelly hemostats along the dorsal and ventral extremes of the membrane so that the tips meet at the base of the T cartilage.
10. Cut the membrane along the clamps.
11. Place a third clamp at the base of the T cartilage.
12. Cut the final attachment of the membrane.
13. Leave clamps in place to maintain hemostasis for at least 5 minutes.
14. Remove clamps but do not manipulate eyelids after this.

Superficial lamellar keratectomy

1. Perform general anesthesia.
2. Clip and prep eye.
3. Make an incision around the lesion.

   In the cornea, this should penetrate the epithelium and the superficial stroma, but not so deep as to puncture the anterior chamber. When done correctly, the wound edges should relax and part slightly.

   In the conjunctiva (for lesions that extend this far) use tenotomy scissors.
4. Elevate the corneal wound edge using small tissue forceps.
5. Separate the superficial stroma using corneal dissectors, this should be rotated carefully and advance easily. If the lesion extends into the conjunctiva, tenotomy scissors will be required for this portion and bleeding is likely; this can be managed with gentle pressure.
6. Check wound bed to ensure complete removal of the lesion.
7. Final steps for more complicated lesions include the following:

   For deeper lesions, a conjunctival flap maybe required.

   For lesions that extend into the conjunctiva, the conjunctival edge should be anchored to the limbus using an absorbable suture with a simple continuous pattern.

Postoperative care

Ciliary muscle spasm can be inhibited using atropine 2 or 3 times a day with topical antibiotics.

Inspect daily, paying particular attention to infection, malacia, and corneal stability.

Recheck in 1 week, small lesions should no longer retain a fluorescein stain; larger lesions may take 2 weeks.

Removal of the retrobulbar fat pad

1. Make a small incision into and through the conjunctiva.
2. Excise the fat.
3. Close the incision with a small absorbable suture.

Box 3
Protecting ulcers

Membrana nictitans or third eyelid flaps

1. Gently stretch the nictitans membrane across the surface of the cornea to establish which direction it normally moves.

2. Suture the free edge of the membrane to either the dorsal-temporal fornix or the upper lid. Use silk and place 3 horizontal mattress sutures, but do not tighten them.

3. Inspect the bulbar surface of the membrane, it is important that the sutures do not penetrate this surface or severe corneal irritation will occur.

4. Wash the eye to remove mucous, exudates, and debris.

5. Pull the sutures tight in unison. Over tighten the suture if there is tissue swelling because they will loosen when the swelling subsides.

Although these flaps prevent further injury and reduce pain, they also prevent daily examination of the eye. Patients should be observed carefully while the flap is in place, if there is an increase in rubbing, exudate formation, depression, fever, or signs of pain the flap should be removed and the eye reexamined.

Total conjunctival flaps, also known as 360 degrees

1. Dissect the conjunctiva at the limbus, all the way around (hence the name *total* or *360 degrees*).

2. Extend the dissection from the limbus toward the equator of the globe until enough conjunctivas are released that the conjunctiva from the dorsal portion can meet with that of the ventral portion.

3. Use an absorbable suture material and mattress sutures to hold the ventral and dorsal conjunctiva in apposition of the cornea.

This technique does not require corneal sutures to be placed and thus is easier to perform and does not require as much magnification as the others; however, it does tend to result in a more opaque scar.

Conjunctival flaps: pedicle

1. Dissect a flap of conjunctiva parallel to, and at least 2 mm away from, the limbus. The size of graft required depends on the size of the ulcer to be covered. To preserve blood supply, it is advised that the base of the graft is slightly wider than the free end.

2. Cover the graft with a moist sterile swab.

3. Remove all necrotic tissue and debris from the defect (eg, the ulcer).

4. Suture the free end of the graft to the cornea using absorbable suture material and simple interrupted sutures. Sutures should be placed through the graft first, then pass through the damaged cornea to exit the normal cornea.

5. Close the paralimbal wound using absorbable suture material and a continuous pattern.

6. After the defects have healed, the graft can be cut using tenotomy scissors.

Paralysis of the palpebral nerve is usually caused by trauma and results in a unilateral or bilateral inability to blink the eyelid. As mentioned previously, the eyelid performs 2 essential roles in ocular health, both of which are diminished if it cannot move. Thus, paralysis of the palpebral nerve leaves the cornea susceptible to exposure keratitis, corneal ulceration, and hyperkeratosis. If topical medications cannot be administered frequently enough to compensate for this, then a membrana nictitans flap (see **Box 3**) or temporary tarsorrhaphy is indicated (see **Box 4**). A reversible

---

Box 4
Tarsorrhaphy

Temporary tarsorrhaphy

1. Sedate the patient.

2. Perform local and topical anesthesia.

3. Thread a nonabsorbable suture material through a stent.

4. Enter the eyelid skin approximately 5 mm from the upper eyelid margin and exit through the hairless portion of the eyelid margin. Make sure that the suture does not penetrate the tarsal plate or conjunctiva at any point.

5. Pass the suture into the lower eyelid through the hairless portion of the margin and exit through the skin approximately 5 mm from the margin.

6. Pass the suture through another stent.

7. Repeat steps 3 to 6 going from the lower lid to the upper lid.

8. Repeat steps 3 to 7 to place as many sutures as desired.

9. Tighten the sutures.

10. Knot the tightened sutures. If access to the eye is required (for example to allow examination later), these can be bowed knots but care must be taken to ensure that the ends do not irritate the cornea.

Reversible split-lid tarsorrhaphy

1. Restrain the patient either by general anesthesia or heavy sedation and local anesthesia.

2. Use a scalpel blade to split the eyelids by incising into the eyelid margin following the tarsal gland orifices. Incision should be approximately 6-mm deep and 6-mm wide and split the eyelid into an outer layer composed of the skin and orbicularis muscle, and the other layer containing the tarsal plate and conjunctiva. Place one incision central in the upper eyelid and one centrally in the lower lid, and then also place incisions in the temporal third of both lids.

3. Place an absorbable suture into the base of the upper eyelid split and then into the base of the lower eyelid split.

4. Tighten the suture and tie a knot. This procedure will cause the outer layers to meet and move externally while the inner layers meet and push toward the cornea, burying the knot within the middle.

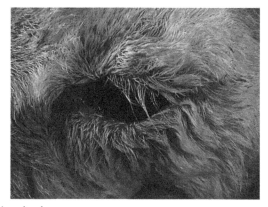

Fig. 2. Entropion in a lamb.

> **Box 5**
> **Entropion correction**
>
> In valuable animals, entropion can be corrected as it is in small animals by using the Hotz-Celsus procedure. However, for simpler cases where a saline injection has not been successful, the entropion can be corrected using horizontal mattress tacking sutures, staples, or clips.
>
> 1. The Hotz-Celsus procedure removes a thin elliptical section of skin and orbicularis oculi muscle from the lid. The length, width, and shape of the section should be determined preoperatively.
>
> 2. Incise the skin and orbicularis oculi muscle about 1 to 2 mm away from the margin, continue the incision parallel to the margin, and form the ellipse by making the lower incision slightly arch shaped.
>
> 3. Dissect the elliptical strip of skin and orbicularis oculi muscle carefully and excise using tenotomy scissors.
>
> 4. Suture the wound using diverging, simple interrupted sutures to accommodate the two different lengths of the wound edges.

split-lid tarsorrhaphy is recommended for cases where return of eyelid function is not expected to occur within a few weeks.

Tumors involving the eyelid are more common in cattle than other farmed species. Benign papillomas, thought to be of viral origin, and locally aggressive squamous cell carcinomas are both common. When small wartlike lesions are present on small ruminants, it is important to rule out the zoonotic disease contagious ecthyma. Which therapeutic approach you take depends on both the value and intended use of the animal as well as the size and progression of the lesion. Lesions affecting the eyelid margin, or large enough to irritate the eye, need to be removed. Because squamous cell carcinomas are aggressive, the earlier the treatment can be initiated the less invasive it is likely to be, but that many small lesions (< 3 mm) may spontaneously regress.[5] Small lesions less than 1 cm may be removed by sharp excision; larger lesions may require tent-shaped excision or H blepharoplasty (see **Box 2**).[6] Other therapies, including cryosurgery,[7] radiofrequency hyperthermia, and immunotherapy, have been used.

The Nictitating Membrane

The nictitating membrane, commonly known as the third eyelid, can suffer from squamous cell carcinomas, lacerations, trauma resulting in exposure of the cartilage,

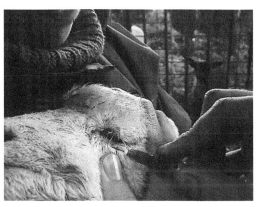

Fig. 3. Lamb entropion resolved by intrapalpebral injection of long-acting antibiotic depot.

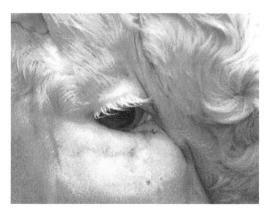

Fig. 4. Entropion in a Charolais bull.

orbital fat prolapse and, in sheep and goats, follicular hyperplasia. Unlike cats and dogs who rely on the secretions of the membrana nictitans glands to prevent desiccation of the eye, cattle and other large animals appear to do fine without it[8]; thus where repair is not possible, excision can be performed without comprising ocular health (**Fig. 6**).

The Cornea

An ocular dermoid[9] is a skinlike lesion on the cornea, conjunctiva, sclera, or eyelid (**Fig. 7**A). This condition is congenital; although they may be asymptomatic at birth

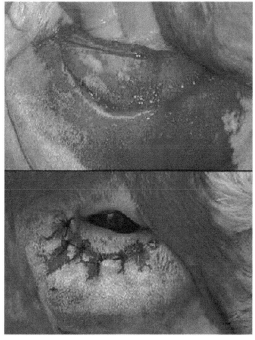

Fig. 5. Surgery with the Hotz-Celsus technique. Excision of a sizeable portion of eyelid skin using the Hotz-Celsus technique was curative.

Box 6
Repair of lacerations

Eyelid lacerations

1. Give antibiotics before surgery.

2. Sedate or perform general anesthesia, depending on the temperament of the animal.

3. Prepare lid by repeated povidone iodine cleaning and sterile water rinses. This stage may also involve clipping any hair on the lid, if so, place a sterile gel on the wound to prevent contamination by tiny hair but be sure to wash this gel away thoroughly before operating.

4. Check for foreign bodies.

5. Debride as little as possible. Every bit of eyelid tissue, especially the margin, is important for correct function and even that which appears badly damaged and beyond hope may heal well. For wounds less than 24 hours old, rubbing with a piece of dry gauze until the wound bleeds is sufficient debridement.

6. Close in 3 layers using absorbable sutures in a figure-of-8 pattern. The deep layer includes the tarsal plate and ought to contain the orbicularis oculi muscle. The middle layer should be placed in the subcuticular tissues. The final layer is placed in the skin, which can be closed routinely. The first suture is the most important and must result in perfect alignment and apposition of the wound and eyelid margin. If the wound is severe, a stent should be used to aid support of the lid.

7. Postoperative care should include warm compresses as well as topical antibiotics and corticosteroids.

Globe lacerations

1. Advise the owner before your arrival not to touch the eye and to prevent, where possible, any self-trauma by the animal. No ointment or other topical medication should be applied; this is also true during surgery.

2. Sedate the patient, paralyze the eyelid, and then examine.

3. Perform general anesthesia. Protect the eye during induction.

4. Prepare the surgical field and then take a swab for culture.

5. Lavage the eye gently.

6. Replace the healthy uveal tissue into the anterior chamber.

7. Excise the necrotic, damaged, or obviously contaminated tissue. Uveal tissue will bleed, which can be managed using microcautery.

8. Irrigate the anterior chamber using lactated Ringer or balanced salt solution.

9. Close wound. It is important that the two edges appose each other exactly. Sutures should be placed deep but must not penetrate the basement membrane. Begin the suture by entering the cornea perpendicular to its surface and then exit the other side in the same manner.

10. Reform the chamber by inserting an 18-guage needle through the limbus and instilling the lactated ringers or balanced salt solution.

11. Check the wound integrity by applying fluorescein stain and gentle pressure to the globe.

12. Place a transpalpebral lavage device (see previous discussion).

---

they disrupt distribution of the tear film, cause chronic irritation, and impair vision. Most dermoids do not extend beyond the corneal epithelium and should be removed by careful superficial lamellar keratectomy (see **Fig. 7**B) (see **Box 2**).

Whenever the cornea or sclera is lacerated, the prognosis is guarded. For those lacerations that are not full thickness, where the anterior chamber is still formed and

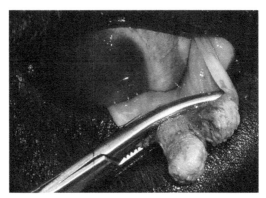

Fig. 6. Nictitating membrane clamped before removal of marginal mass.

contains minimal hemorrhage or fibrin, the prognosis is slightly better. Bearing this in mind, it is advisable to discuss enucleation or intrascleral prosthesis placement as an alternative to surgery. However, heavily contaminated lacerations are not suitable for prosthesis placement. If the lens has also ruptured it should be dealt with by

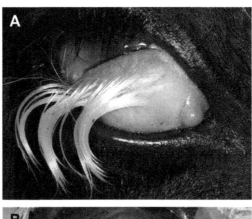

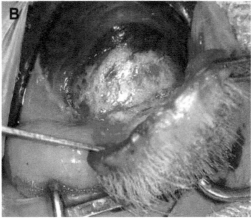

Fig. 7. (*A*) An ocular dermoid. (*B*) Corneoconjunctival dermoid in a calf and its removal by superficial keratectomy. (*Courtesy of* Dr D.A. Ward, University of Tennessee, Department of Small Animal Clinical Sciences, Veterinary Teaching Hospital, Knoxville, TN.)

phacoemulsification. Surgical repair is required immediately for full-thickness lacerations or those where the wound margins are separated by more than 2 to 3 mm. General anesthesia, magnification, and appropriate ophthalmic instruments are essential for such procedures and thus it is usually better to refer such cases to a specialist.

Foreign bodies cause pain and discomfort and need to be completely removed as soon as possible. The depth of a foreign body should always be assessed carefully, and extreme caution applied when investigating black foreign bodies in the cornea as these may actually be a piece of iris or corpora nigra sealing a perforation. Large, deep, penetrating foreign bodies and suspected perforations are best referred to a specialist who is capable of managing a perforation for removal under general anesthesia. More superficial bodies can often be removed with a spray of sterile saline.

Large or deep corneal ulcers can benefit from surgical intervention in addition to medical management. Third eyelid flaps provide protection and support, reducing pain and preventing further injury, but can be aesthetically unpleasing and hinder monitoring. Conjunctival flaps bring a blood supply to the area providing the ulcer with blood components, fibrovascular tissue to support the wound, and also increase the concentration of drugs given systemically. Many techniques for conjunctival flaps have been described and will be discussed later. When performing any of these, it is important to remember that despite their obvious advantages to healing, they leave a permanent scar, which can be dense and impair vision. If a trained veterinary surgeon, operating microscopes, and special instruments are available, then corneal ulcers can also be treated by corneoscleral transposition, lamellar keratoplasty, and penetrating keratoplasty.

Cataracts[10,11] are rare in farm animals compared with small pets and horses. If removal is necessary, then phacoemulsification should be performed. Phacoemulsification uses high-frequency ultrasound to fragment the lens. Normal pressure is maintained within the anterior chamber through irrigation, and then suction is used to remove the fragments and the irrigation fluid.

BEFORE SURGERY
Considerations Before Surgery

Several decisions need to be made by the veterinarian and the owner before embarking on a surgical procedure. Firstly, a thorough examination of the whole animal must be performed, followed by a detailed ophthalmologic examination (see the article on Clinical Examination elsewhere in this issue for further exploration of this topic); this is to provide a diagnosis for the problem and determine the extent of the disease. This information in turn can be used to decide appropriate options for therapy and compare the relative prognosis and outcome for each option. At this point it is important to discuss with the owner what they are looking for in terms of outcome and how much they are willing to spend. This information will vary depending on the age of the animal, its pregnancy status (if female), its purpose, and its economic and potentially sentimental value. For example, on a beef breeding farm with a cow in late pregnancy, it may be more important that she survives to deliver the calf; however, if the same condition was present in the best show bull, then aesthetic appearance may be more important. Whatever the constraints and desired outcome, it remains important that animal welfare is considered and not compromised.

Once a surgical procedure has been agreed, 3 more important choices remain to be decided: (1) who is going to perform the surgery (some of the more complicated and delicate surgery is better performed by a specialist who has more facilities, equipment and experience), (2) where to perform the surgery (eg, in the field or a hospital setting), and (3) what type of anesthesia will be used (standing under sedation or under full general anesthesia).

Materials

Irby suggests that a basic ophthalmic instrument set should contain the items listed in **Box 7**.

Silk can be used for stay sutures; whereas, synthetic absorbable suture material should be used for ligation and subcutaneous procedures. Corneal repair requires fine absorbable suture material and the smallest available needle size should be used. The skin can be closed with a nonabsorbable suture; the exact pattern will depend on the procedure performed and the surgeon's own preference (eg, simple interrupted following entropion correction or ford interlocking after an enucleation).

Preparing For Surgery

For surgery to be feasible it will be necessary to restrain patients. Good restraint is essential for the safety of both the patients and the humans involved. It is also

---

Box 7
Surgical Instruments for Ophthalmic Surgery

Small towel clamps

#9 blade handle

Small mayo scissors

General suture scissors

Small stitch scissors

Large curved utility scissors with serrated blade

Small curved Metzenbaum scissors

Small straight Metzenbaum scissors

Small ophthalmic scissors

Adson forceps

Allis tissue forceps

Bishop-Harmon fine forceps

Small tissue forceps suitable for conjunctiva or cornea

Snellen or Desmarres lid forceps with solid lower plate

Hartman curved mosquito hemostats (4 pairs)

Kelly hemostats (4 pairs)

Small needle holder

Small needle holder suitable for sutures smaller than 5-0

Curved Castroviejo needle holder

Double-ended Martinez corneal dissector

Eyelid speculum

Desmarres lid retractors (2)

Nonlinting sponges

important because surgery requires precision, and this is much easier if the patients are still. Restraint can be achieved manually by use of a head collar, crush, or chute. Sedation is commonly used to aid restraint, but for those procedures where good restraint is imperative, then general anesthesia can be used.

Before-, during-, and after-surgery steps must be taken to protect the eye. In the normal eye, blinking of the eyelids spreads the tear film across the cornea. The tear film is important because it prevents the cornea from drying out. During surgery the eyelids will be open, so this natural protection is lost and it is important that we take steps to compensate. The easiest way to do this is by using sterile tear preparations; however, if intraocular surgery is planned, then the use of corneal ointments should not occur. As an alternative measure, the eyelids should be closed regularly and sterile saline should be applied.

Considering the preparation of the periocular tissues brings us to the debate about clipping hair. Hair is a source of contamination in any surgical field; as with most surgeries, it could be assumed that we should remove it to minimize the risk of contamination. However, it is possible that clipping may result in small pieces of hair becoming trapped in the conjunctival follicles and not removed at rinsing resulting in increased contamination of the surgical site. Some surgeons prefer to clip only long and dirty hairs carefully with scissors, to remove obvious gross contamination while ensuring that all cut hair is removed. The other concern regarding clipping is that the use of electrical clipping may damage and irritate the eye or periocular tissues, which can be avoided by ensuring the clipper blades are sharp and exercising extreme care when performing the clip. If it is decided that clipping is necessary, then it is vital that all pieces of hair are removed, paying particular attention to the conjunctival sac, which requires repeated flushing. Repeated flushes are beneficial before surgery even if clipping has not occurred because it removes debris from the nasolacrimal duct, which could enter during surgery. Clipping is the preferred method for hair removal despite the disadvantages previously discussed. Chemical depilatories or waves should not be used because they cause swelling and irritation.

To disinfect the surrounding tissues, 10% povidone iodine in sterile water should be used. As with preparation of any site, repeated cleaning should be performed starting from the center, in this case the eyelid margins, circling outwards. The spiral should move out from the center distally and no swab used distally should ever then touch a more central site. Surgical detergents should not be used because there is a risk that they may cause irritation.

Drapes are not usually used in the field; however, in the hospital, if the surgeon wishes to uses drapes, there are many different kinds available from cotton to self-adhesive and all are suitable.

Anesthesia

In addition to restraint, sedation, and either local or general anesthesia is necessary to perform ocular surgery. Xylazine, either alone or in combination with butorphanol, is commonly used in food animals.[12] A dose much lower than that used in horses is recommended (0.1 mg/kg or less intravenously). When sedating cattle, always be aware that recumbency may occur and ensure that bystanders are safe and that the method of restraint will not harm the patients, should this occur. In late gestation, xylazine can cause abortion.

Although general anesthesia can be useful for severe lesions, delicate surgery, or for animals that cannot be adequately restrained or sedated otherwise, it is usually not necessary because most ocular techniques can be performed using a variety of local anesthesia methods.

An auriculopalpebral local anesthetic block inhibits motor signals to eyelids producing akinesia but does not provide any analgesia. Therefore, although this is useful to allow access to the eye, it is necessary to combine this with other techniques to prevent sensory appreciation of pain. A total of 5 to 6 mL of 2% lidocaine should be injected caudal to the lateral canthus into the subcutaneous tissue along the dorsal axis of the zygomatic arch approximately 5-cm caudal to the frontal process of the zygomatic bone.

There are multiple options for providing analgesia to the eye, and these are described in various textbooks.[13] Each block has its own advantages and disadvantages and with any block there is the risk of toxicity, trauma, or incorrect placement. The choice of block is usually based on the surgeon's own preference and experience, bearing in mind the disease and procedure to be performed.

The Peterson block blocks the oculomotor, trochlear, and abducens nerves as well as the ophthalmic, maxillary, and mandibular branches of the trigeminal where they exit the foramen orbitorotundum. It is commonly used to provide analgesia to the eye and orbit as well as immobilization of the globe; however, it does not block the eyelids.

The alternatives to a Peterson block are the single-point or 4-point retrobulbar block. These alternatives are thought to be easier to perform but carry a greater risk of orbital hemorrhage, direct pressure on the globe, penetration of the globe, damage to the optic nerve, or injection into the optic nerve meninges. Again, the technique for performing these blocks is described in other textbooks and articles.

Neither the Peterson nor the retrobulbar block will provide sufficient analgesia of the eyelids, so it is recommended that these blocks are used in combination with a ring block. Here, 5 to 10 mL of lidocaine can be injected subcutaneously around the eyelid margins.

Perioperative Management

Antiinflammatories given preoperatively have been shown to reduce the need for postoperative pain relief and they help prevent the wind-up phenomena associated with pain. Schulz suggests that 1 mg/kg of flunixin meglumine given intravenously immediately before surgery is sufficient for enucleations procedures. Although, obviously the extent of both the disease process and the excision should be taken into account when choosing a dose.

If operating in a field, as many will be, the risk of infection is high. To prevent this from occurring, a surgeon should give systemic broad spectrum antibiotics in addition to following the general rules of surgical asepsis.

AFTER SURGERY
Postoperative Care

After surgery the eye needs to heal; this will happen best if self-trauma by patients can be prevented. Membrane flaps and tarsorrhaphies, as previously described can help but are contraindicated in some instances as discussed in globe lacerations. They also prevent observation of the eye which is also important to monitor healing and any complications that may arise. In cases where infection is suspected or confirmed then antibiotics may be give post operatively, where necessary; this was mentioned in the relevant technique description. Application of topical medication can be challenging in food animals, a transpalpebral ocular lavage system can make this a lot easier (**Box 8**).[14] Where nonabsorbable sutures are used to close the skin these should be removed and the area reexamined 10 to 14 days after suture, or sooner if complications occur.

Box 8
Transpalpebral catheter placement

1. Sedate the patient.

2. Prepare the skin over the dorsolateral orbital rim.

3. Paralyze the upper eyelid using a nerve block of choice and inject local anesthetic subcutaneously.

4. Prepare the tubing by fixing within a hubless needle or to a wound-drain insertion needle.

5. Hold the needle with the tip against the index finger and tubing held in the palm of the hand. Place the fingernail toward the cornea.

6. Rest the needle tip on orbital rim.

7. Pull the upper eyelid away from the globe over the needle.

8. Advance the needle tip through the upper eyelid. Take care not to trap any fold of conjunctiva at this stage.

9. Pull the tubing gently so the footplate rests in the conjunctiva sac.

10. Check that the eyelid moves freely.

11. Secure the tubing, place small pieces of tape around the tubing where it exits the eyelid and spaced out more distally, then suture these to the skin. Cyanoacrylate glue can also be applied for extra security.

Complications

As with any surgery, after eye surgery there is always the risk of infection and wound dehiscence. If the surgery has been performed to remove a neoplastic lesion, then the risk of incomplete removal and progression of the neoplasia is always present. Owners should be made aware of this before surgery, and steps should be taken to minimize this risk during surgery by aiming for clean margins and using a clean blade for each cut to prevent spreading neoplastic cells.

SUMMARY

Although medical management of eye conditions is common place, surgical therapy is possible, achievable, and advisable for many conditions. Many of these techniques can be performed in the field and, when approached correctly, can have positive outcomes for animal welfare, health, and productivity.

REFERENCES

1. Rebhun WC. Ocular manifestations of systemic diseases in cattle. Vet Clin North Am Large Anim Pract 1984;6(3):623–39.
2. Rebhum WC. Diseases of the bovine orbit and globe. J Am Vet Med Assoc 1979; 175:171–5.
3. Vermunt J. Transpalpebral exenteration in cattle. Vet Q 1984;6(1):46–8.
4. Lamprecht H, Pfeiffer A. Entropion in newborn lambs. Berl Munch Tierarztl Wochenschr 1989;102(9):303–10.
5. Sloss V, Smith TJ, De Yi G. Controlling ocular squamous cell carcinoma in Hereford cattle. Aust Vet J 1986;63(8):248–51.
6. Welker B, Modransky PD, Hoffsis GF, et al. Excision of neoplasms of the bovine lower eyelid by H-blepharoplasty. Vet Surg 1992;20(2):133–9.

7. Farris HE, Fraunfelder FT. Cryosurgical treatment of ocular squamous cell carcinoma of cattle. J Am Vet Med Assoc 1976;168(3):213–6.

8. Irby NL. Surgical diseases of the eye in farm animals. In: Fubini SL, Ducharme NG, editors. Farm animal surgery. St Louis (MO): Saunders; 2004.

9. Barkyoumb SD, Leipold HW. Nature and cause of bilateral ocular dermoid in Hereford cattle. Vet Pathol 1984;21(3):316–24.

10. Gionfriddo JR, Blair M. Congenital and persistent hyaloids vasculature in a llama. Vet Ophthalmol 2002;5(1):65–70.

11. Oz HH, McClure RJ, Hillman DJ. Bilateral cataract surgery in a Suffolk ewe. Vet Rec 1986;118(18):512–3.

12. Schulz K. Field surgery of the eye and para-orbital tissues. Vet Clin North Am Food Anim Pract 2008;24:527–34.

13. Muir WW, Hubbell AE. Local anaesthesia in cattle, sheep, goats and pigs. In: Handbook of veterinary anaesthesia. Mosby;2007.

14. Severin GA. Severin's veterinary ophthalmology notes. 3rd edition. Fort Collins (CO): Veterinary Ophthalmology Notes; 1996.

Congenital Abnormalities in Production Animals

David L. Williams, MA, VetMB, PhD, CertVOphthal, CertWEL, FRCVS

KEYWORDS

• Ruminant • Congenital • Eye • Microphthalmia

The increase in number of food-producing animals raised each year implies that even small prevalences of congenital anomalies in these ruminant species are still reflected in a significant number of affected animals born each year. The problem for an ophthalmologist interested in such conditions is accessing these animals. Most animals with a spontaneous idiopathic condition present as a single case in a farm population and are normally euthanized and disposed of without even alerting the veterinarian responsible for the flock or herd, let alone a specialist in a referral institution situated at some distance from the farm. It takes a specific investigation, such as that of Hässig and colleagues[1] into the association between congenital bovine cataract and electric power lines, to show the true incidence of such congenital abnormalities. Although insufficient, such studies are currently being undertaken to identify the true level of uncommon congenital ocular abnormalities. This article does not provide a complete overview of every congenital eye defect; such overviews are available in the key textbooks of the subject[2,3] and indeed in Leipold's[4] review in the previous issue of the *Veterinary Clinics of North America* on large animal ophthalmology. Rather, this article discusses recent research into several conditions to demonstrate the opportunities that exist for investigating such conditions both from a genetic and an environmental perspective.

ANOPHTHALMOS AND MICROPHTHALMOS

It might seem strange to begin the review of ocular abnormalities with anophthalmos, in which animals are born without eyes. And yet in truth, even when an orbit appears devoid of ocular tissue (**Fig. 1**), almost always a vestigial remnant of ocular tissue can be found; these are cases of extreme microphthalmos. A cattle breed in which anophthalmos is seen as a relatively common disorder is the Japanese brown cow.[5] In this breed, animals are born with a remnant of pigmented tissue deep in the orbit and also with caudal sacral and tail abnormalities. In a study of 921 calves born with bilateral or

Department of Veterinary Medicine, University of Cambridge, Madingley Road, Cambridge CB3 0ES, UK
E-mail address: doctordlwilliams@aol.com

Vet Clin Food Anim 26 (2010) 477–486
doi:10.1016/j.cvfa.2010.09.001
0749-0720/10/$ – see front matter © 2010 Elsevier Inc. All rights reserved.

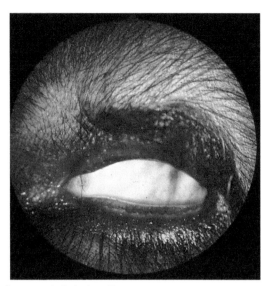

Fig. 1. The orbit of an anophthalmic calf.

unilateral apparent anophthalmos of 231,540 births (giving a prevalence of 0.39%) the authors found that 21% of the animals lacked tail or had other severe sacral abnormalities (**Fig. 2**). In humans, this so-called anophthalmia-plus syndrome has been reported,[6] but the embryologic link between globe development and caudal vertebral abnormalities is unclear. The orbit in any anophthalmic animal or human fails to develop normally because the normally enlarging globe regulates the development of the surrounding bony structures. Thus anophthalmic or severely microphthalmic animals have abnormally small orbits (**Fig. 3**).

It is known that genetic mutations of the homeobox pax 6 gene, the master control gene of the eye,[7] lead to aniridia when in the heterozygous state and anophthalmos when homozygous.[8] In fact, later work has shown a cascade of gene products necessary for normal globe development, with sine oculis and eyes absent activated by the eyeless gene product[9] and vax2 mediating the activation or inhibition of pax 6, with sonic hedgehog modulating the position of the vax2 gene product in the nucleus or cytoplasm.[10] With such a complex interaction of genes, it is not surprising that the

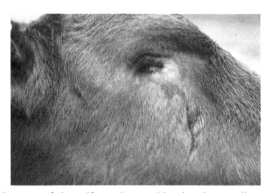

Fig. 2. The facial features of the calf are distorted by the abnormally small orbit.

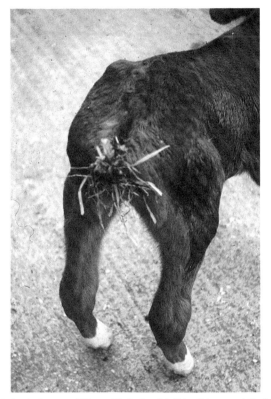

Fig. 3. Caudal vertebral abnormalities with lack of tail in this anophthalmic calf.

mutation responsible for anophthalmos in Japanese brown cattle or the sporadic cases seen rarely in the United Kingdom and Europe have not been identified.

Indeed, environmental factors may also play an important part. Vitamin A is essential not only in retinal function when the eye is fully developed but also in eye development itself, as described in later sections.[11] Piglets born with hypovitaminosis A have been reported to have abnormalities in globe development.[12,13] Attempts were made to link the birth of clusters of offsprings with anophthalmos to the use of the fungicide benzimidazole (Benomyl),[14] which can cause the developmental defect in rats [15] Indeed, this was the reason for the epidemiologic study in bovine anophthalmos by the author. Evidence is lacking for a link in humans or cattle.

Microphthalmos in sheep, manifested as clinical anophthalmos, with an apparently empty orbit (**Fig. 4**), was first noted in New Zealand[16] and has since been intricately studied through a collaborative effort by researchers in Switzerland, Germany, and Australia. The condition occurs as an autosomal recessive trait and has been linked to a region on chromosome 23[17] involving a missense mutation in the homeobox gene PITX3.[18] Such detailed work allows the condition to be used as a model for similar pathologic condition in man.

CYCLOPIA

A well-recognized abnormality is cyclopia in the offspring of sheep feeding on the corn lily *Veratrum californicum* (**Fig. 5**).

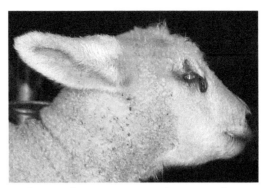

Fig. 4. Microphthalmic lamb with PITX3 mutation. (*Courtesy of* Dr C. Drögemüller, Berne, Switzerland.)

The condition was first noted in Idaho in the late 1950s in sheep grazing in fields containing this plant. The development of cyclopia, in which one frontal eye exists (see **Fig. 5**), or synophthalmia, in which both eyes are joined in one frontal orbit (see **Fig. 2**A in the article by Middleton elsewhere in this issue), is part of a wide range of craniofacial abnormalities arising from the teratogenic action of the alkaloidal steroid cyclopamine,[19,20] but with a relatively narrow window of activity, both temporally and dose-related.[21] Cyclopamine inhibits the hedgehog signal transduction pathway. Mouse embryos cultured in the presence of cyclopamine to silence their sonic hedgehog gene show these changes of cyclopia and the associated developmental brain defect holoprosencephaly.[22] Given that the sonic hedgehog gene is involved

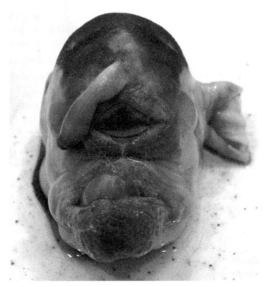

Fig. 5. A cyclopic lamb born by cesarean delivery at 135 days' gestation. Note the single central eye and the proboscis characteristic of such developmental defects. (*Courtesy of* Poisonous Plant Research Laboratory, Agricultural Research Service, United States Department of Agriculture, Logan, UT.)

in several cancers, cyclopamine may be a valuable antineoplastic agent.[23] The condition can be avoided by preventing pregnant sheep from ingesting the lilies. Whereas the teratogens produce craniofacial defects and microphthalmia in laboratory rodents, cyclopia is not a well-recognized consequence of administration.[24]

MULTIPLE CONGENITAL ANOMALIES: GENETIC AND INFECTIOUS CAUSES

A syndrome of iris and lens defects, microphthalmia, retained embryonic intraocular vasculature, and retinal dysplasia and detachment has been reported in cattle for nearly 40 years.[25–27] But it is only in the last one year that the genetic mutation responsible for this apparently diverse set of lesions has been discovered.[28] The WFDC gene on chromosome 18 encodes a small secretory protein, which acts as a protease inhibitor, and in Japanese black cattle with recessively inherited multiple congenital ocular defects, a frameshift mutation prematurely terminates gene expression. However, not all cattle have a recessively inherited trait, and linkage analysis has also shown a dominantly inherited gene mutation on chromosome 5, which accounts for the genetic heterogeneity of the condition.[29]

Other nongenetic etiologic factors can be associated with multiple congenital ocular defects. Of these, a key one is hypovitaminosis A during fetal development. In one report, microphthalmos, microcornea, aphakia, absence of iridal structures with retinal dysplasia, and a degree of optic nerve hypoplasia were noted in 25% of calves born to a group of suckler cows, which themselves showed signs of vitamin deficiency, such as blindness and papilledema.[30] A more recent article from France reported that cows with similar signs and a similar history of maternal malnutrition produced calves with microphthalmia, aphakic globes with retinal dysplasia, and optic nerve hypoplasia.[31]

An important infectious cause of ocular deformities in cattle is the pestivirus bovine viral diarrhea.[32] Retinitis resulting form viral infection leads to retinal dysplasia,[33] whereas other defects can include cataract and more profound developmental globe abnormalities.[34] Exposure of the dam to such infection between 125 to 175 days of gestation can lead to these ocular birth defects together with neurologic abnormalities, whereas exposure after 175 days typically leads to a healthy calf fully immune at birth.[35]

Another viral infection, emerging in the United Kingdom and Europe as a consequence of the northerly spread of the transmitting midges, is the orbivirus bluetongue. Although not causing globe defects, intrauterine infection of the developing calf or lamb by the virus can lead to hydrencephaly with complete lack of the cerebral hemispheres.[36,37] These animals, while still having a pupillary light reflex, because their midbrain is still present and functioning, are behaviorally blind and are noted to be "dummy" calves. Profound corneal edema has also been reported in some calves infected in utero with bluetongue virus,[38] although these calves were not affected by hydrencephaly (**Fig. 6**).

CONGENITAL CATARACT

Congenital cataracts have been documented in cattle in several reports, with the prevalence as high as 34% in some herds.[39] In a large study in England undertaken as a doctoral study by Caroline Manser (née Cley),[39] 3.7% of more than 800 calves were noted to have lens opacities (**Fig. 7**). While it was impossible to assign a specific cause to lens opacities, they were seen in calves born later in the summer months and were rarely seen in heifers. Cataracts linked to genetic defects generally include other ocular abnormalities such as retinal detachment, aniridia, microphakia, and

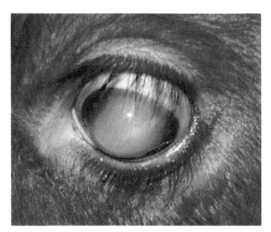

Fig. 6. Profound corneal edema in a calf infected with bluetongue virus.

hydrocephalus. As discussed earlier, microphthalmia and cataracts with retinal dysplasia have been documented in calves exposed to bovine viral diarrhea in utero.

Manser's doctoral studies were undertaken in the late 1970s, and since then little new work has been reported until last year when Hässig and colleagues[1] published a study potentially linking nuclear cataract in Swiss veal calves with mobile telephone antennae. On 1 farm, a quarter of newborn calves had lens opacities. In a randomized study, slightly more than 250 veal calves from Swiss abattoirs were examined, their proximity of birth to mobile telephone base station antennae was determined, and samples were taken to evaluate signs of infectious agents, such as bovine viral diarrhea, *Toxoplasma*, and *Neospora*, and to document signs of oxidative stress. Oxidative stress is a key feature of many forms of cataract, with oxidation causing cross-linking of thiol groups of lens crystallins with subsequent protein aggregation and cataract formation.[40,41] Of 156 male calves, 37% had cataract, whereas 25% of female calves showed lens opacities. The association between cataract and proximity to telephone mast and electromagnetic field strength was statistically significant, as was the association between cataract and intraocular oxidative stress as determined by the concentration of the protective antioxidant enzymes superoxide dismutase, catalase, and glutathione peroxidase.[1] It remains for others to investigate the extent to which electromagnetic radiation from mobile telephone mast is associated

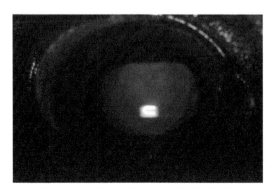

Fig. 7. Nuclear cataract. (*Courtesy of* Dr C. Manser (née Cley), Histon, Cambridge.)

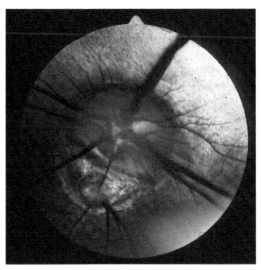

Fig. 8. A typical (ie, at 6-o'clock position) coloboma in a Charolais bull.

with nuclear cataracts in calves. Clearly, there must be other etiologic factors, mobile telephones were not in existence in the 1970s when Caroline Cley published her thesis, and anecdotal comments suggest that an association between marshy environments and these nuclear cataracts may exist (Scott D, personal communication, 2010).

OPTIC NERVE COLOBOMAS

Optic nerve coloboma (**Fig. 8**) was first described in Charolais cattle by Barnett and Ogien[42] in 1972 and subsequently reported by others also.[43] The genetics of these lesions is somewhat curious: the autosomal dominant inheritance of the condition is completely penetrant in the bull but only incompletely penetrant (52%) in the cow, whereas it is apparently recessive in F1 crossbred animals.[44] The condition is still prevalent in the breed, with the author having seen several herds with significant numbers of animals affected, as might be expected in a dominantly inherited trait, but a condition not obvious unless the eye is specifically examined with an ophthalmo-scope. Animals do not seem to be particularly affected with regard to their vision, although clear assessment of bovine visual acuity is not readily accomplished in a farm environment. Whereas developmental defects of the optic nerve in humans are often associated with other ocular signs related to failure of optic cup closure,[45] neurologic abnormalities,[46] or genetic systemic disorders,[47] none of these seem to occur in these Charolais cattle. The colobomas are certainly associated with an abnor-mality in optic cup fissure closure, as demonstrated by their predominantly typical (ie ventral) appearance (see **Fig. 8**), but this occurs with the formation of a cystic defect, as often seen in optic nerve colobomas in other species.[48,49]

SUMMARY

The substantial volume of research into congenital defects in ruminants means that a review such as this can only skim the surface of the subject. Whole books could be written with an article for each condition. Indeed, this author has not touched on many interesting areas such as dermoids in cattle or ocular neoplasms seen at or shortly after birth. Nevertheless, it is hoped that the information presented in this article has shown the great advances that have been made in many areas, at least regarding the etiology and pathogenesis of several conditions since Leipold's[4] review. Emerging diseases such as bluetongue need further work. Although Osburn's paper from 1972[37] shows that this is hardly a new disease, it is just one newly presenting to us in the cold North as the world warms. Human interventions from Benomyl and its potential involvement with anophthalmos to mobile phone microwave radiation and bovine cataract are likely to expand in years to come and may render the field of congenital eye disease in farm animals even more important than it is at present.

REFERENCES

1. Hässig M, Jud F, Naegeli H, et al. Prevalence of nuclear cataract in Swiss veal calves and its possible association with mobile telephone antenna base stations. Schweiz Arch Tierheilkd 2009;151:471–8.
2. Townsend WM. Food and fiber-producing animal ophthalmology. In: Gelatt KN. Veterinary ophthalmology. 4th edition. Oxford (UK): Blackwell Publishing; 2007. p. 1275–335.
3. Lavach JD. Large animal ophthalmology. St Louis (MO): CV Mosby; 1990.
4. Leipold HW. Congenital ocular defects in food-producing animals. Vet Clin North Am Large Anim Pract 1984;6:577–95.
5. Moritomo Y, Koga O, Miyamoto H, et al. Congenital anophthalmia with caudal vertebral anomalies in Japanese brown cattle. J Vet Med Sci 1995;57:693–6.
6. Makhoul IR, Soudack M, Kochavi O, et al. Anophthalmia-plus syndrome: a clinical report and review of the literature. Am J Med Genet A 2007;143:64–8.
7. Gehring WJ. The master control gene for morphogenesis and evolution of the eye. Genes Cells 1996;1:11–5.
8. Quiring R, Walldorf U, Kloter U, et al. Homology of the eyeless gene of Drosophila to the Small eye gene in mice and Aniridia in humans. Science 1994;265:785–9.
9. Halder G, Callaerts P, Flister S, et al. Eyeless initiates the expression of both sine oculis and eyes absent during Drosophila compound eye development. Development 1998;125:2181–91.
10. Kim JW, Lemke G. Hedgehog-regulated localization of Vax2 controls eye development. Genes Dev 2006;20:2833–47.
11. Cvekl A, Wang WL. Retinoic acid signaling in mammalian eye development. Exp Eye Res 2009;89:280–91.
12. Palludan B. The influence of vitamin A deficiency on foetal development in pigs with special reference to eye organogenesis. Int J Vitam Nutr Res 1976;46:223–5.
13. Darcel CL, Nilo L, Avery RJ, et al. Microphthalmia and macrophthalmia in piglets. J Pathol Bacteriol 1960;80:281–6.
14. Källén B, Robert E, Harris J. The descriptive epidemiology of anophthalmia and microphthalmia. Int J Epidemiol 1996;25(5):1009–16.
15. Hoogenboom ER, Ransdell JF, Ellis WG, et al. Effects on the fetal rat eye of maternal benomyl exposure and protein malnutrition. Curr Eye Res 1991;10: 601–12.
16. Roe WD, West DM, Walshe MT, et al. Microphthalmia in Texel lambs. N Z Vet J 2003;51:194–5.
17. Tetens J, Ganter M, Müller G, et al. Linkage mapping of ovine microphthalmia to chromosome 23, the sheep orthologue of human chromosome 18. Invest Ophthalmol Vis Sci 2007;48:3506–15.

18. Becker D, Tetens J, Brunner A, et al. Microphthalmia in Texel sheep is associated with a missense mutation in the paired-like homeodomain 3 (PITX3) gene. PLoS One 2010;5:e8689.

19. Bryden MM, Evans HE, Keeler RF. Cyclopia in sheep caused by plant teratogens. J Anat 1971;110:507.

20. Keeler RF. Cyclopamine and related steroidal alkaloid teratogens: their occurrence, structural relationship, and biologic effects. Lipids 1978;13:708–15.

21. Welch KD, Panter KE, Lee ST, et al. Cyclopamine-induced synophthalmia in sheep: defining a critical window and toxicokinetic evaluation. J Appl Toxicol 2009;29:414–21.

22. Nagase T, Nagase M, Osumi N, et al. Craniofacial anomalies of the cultured mouse embryo induced by inhibition of sonic hedgehog signaling: an animal model of holoprosencephaly. J Craniofac Surg 2005;16:80–8.

23. Berman DM, Karhadkar SS, Hallahan AR, et al. Medulloblastoma growth inhibition by hedgehog pathway blockade. Science 2002;297:1559–61.

24. Keeler RF. Teratogenic effects of cyclopamine and jervine in rats, mice and hamsters. Proc Soc Exp Biol Med 1975;149:302–6.

25. Leipold HW, Gelatt KN, Huston K. Multiple ocular anomalies and hydrocephalus in grade beef Shorthorn cattle. Am J Vet Res 1971;32:1019–26.

26. Rupp GP, Knight AP. Congenital ocular defects in a crossbred beef herd. J Am Vet Med Assoc 1984;184:1149–50.

27. Kaswan RL, Collins LG, Blue JL, et al. Multiple hereditary ocular anomalies in a herd of cattle. J Am Vet Med Assoc 1987;191:97–9.

28. Abbasi AR, Khalaj M, Tsuji T, et al. A mutation of the WFDC1 gene is responsible for multiple ocular defects in cattle. Genomics 2009;94:55–62.

29. Ihara N, Fujita T, Shiga K, et al. Linkage analysis reveals two independent loci for ocular disorders in a local Japanese black cattle population. Anim Genet 2005; 36:132–4.

30. Mason CS, Buxton D, Gartside JF. Congenital ocular abnormalities in calves associated with maternal hypovitaminosis A. Vet Rec 2003;153:213–4.

31. Millemann Y, Benoit-Valiergue H, Bonnin JP, et al. Ocular and cardiac malformations associated with maternal hypovitaminosis A in cattle. Vet Rec 2007;160: 441–3.

32. Bistner SI, Rubin LF, Saunders LZ. The ocular lesions of bovine viral diarrhea-mucosal disease. Pathol Vet 1970;7:275–86.

33. Brown TT, Bistner SI, de Lahunta A, et al. Pathogenetic studies of infection of the bovine fetus with bovine viral diarrhea virus. II. Ocular lesions. Vet Pathol 1975;12: 394–404.

34. Scott FW, Kahrs RF, De Lahunte A, et al. Virus induced congenital anomalies of the bovine fetus. I. Cerebellar degeneration (hypoplasia), ocular lesions and fetal mummification following experimental infection with bovine viral diarrhea-mucosal disease virus. Cornell Vet 1973;63:536–60.

35. Kahrs RF, Scott FW, de Lahunte A. Congenital cerebella hypoplasia and ocular defects in calves following bovine viral diarrhea-mucosal disease infection in pregnant cattle. J Am Vet Med Assoc 1970;156:1443–50.

36. Vercauteren G, Miry C, Vandenbussche F, et al. Bluetongue virus serotype 8-associated congenital hydranencephaly in calves. Transbound Emerg Dis 2008;55:293–8.

37. Osburn BI. Animal model for human disease. Hydranencephaly, porencephaly, cerebral cysts, retinal dysplasia, CNS malformations. Animal model: bluetongue-vaccine-virus infection in fetal lambs. Am J Pathol 1972;67:211–4.

38. Holzhauer M, Vos J. 'Blue eyes' in newborn calves associated with bluetongue infection. Vet Rec 2009;164:403–4.
39. Ashton, Barnett KC, Cley CE. Congenital nuclear cataracts in cattle. Vet Rec 1977;100:505–8.
40. Spector A. Oxidative stress-induced cataract: mechanism of action. FASEB J 1995;9:1173–82.
41. Truscott RJ. Age-related nuclear cataract-oxidation is the key. Exp Eye Res 2005; 80:709–25.
42. Barnett KC, Ogien AL. Ocular colobomata in Charolais cattle. Vet Rec 1972;91: 592.
43. McCormack J. Typical colobomas in Charolais bulls. Vet Med Small Anim Clin 1977;72:1626–8.
44. Falco M, Barnett KC. The inheritance of ocular colobomata in Charolais cattle. Vet Rec 1978;102:102–4.
45. Berk AT, Yaman A, Saatçi AO. Ocular and systemic findings associated with optic disc colobomas. J Pediatr Ophthalmol Strabismus 2003;40:272–8.
46. Golnik KC. Cavitary anomalies of the optic disc: neurologic significance. Curr Neurol Neurosci Rep 2008;8:409–13.
47. Jacobs M, Taylor D. The systemic and genetic significance of congenital optic disc anomalies. Eye (Lond) 1991;5:470–5.
48. Williams DL, Barnett KC. Bilateral optic disc colobomas and microphthalmos in a thoroughbred horse. Vet Rec 1993;132:101–3.
49. Doughty MJ, Sivak JG. Scanning electron microscope evaluation of the corneal endothelium in a case of unilateral microphthalmos with retrobulbar cyst in the pigmented rabbit. Cornea 1993;12:341–7.

Infectious Bovine Keratoconjunctivitis: A Review of Cases in Clinical Practice

Dominic Alexander, BVMS, CBiol, MSB, MRCVS[a,b,*]

KEYWORDS

- Infectious bovine keratoconjunctivitis • Pinkeye
- New forest eye • Cattle • Corneal ulceration

INFECTIOUS BOVINE KERATOCONJUNCTIVITIS: A REVIEW OF CASES

Due to the prominence of the bovine eye, the environments where cattle are kept, and the increasing numbers of animals each stockperson is required to care for, ocular disease is not an infrequent occurrence. Aggression between animals or knocks and bumps during handling and transit can damage the eye. Foreign bodies, such as straw, chaff, and grains of sand, can abrade the cornea. Grazing close to field margins, thorns, barbed wire, and tufts of dry stalks of grass can scratch the cornea too. Rust/corrosion and the sharp drips from galvanized handling systems and penning provide ample opportunity for ocular trauma to occur. All of these physical traumas assist pathogens in penetrating the cornea.

Veterinarians are often called to treat end-stage disease where the eye has been treated, unsuccessfully, before veterinary involvement or the disease has progressed so far that severe, and often irreversible, ocular damage has already occurred and enucleation is the only option.

The accepted principal agent causing disease is the gram-negative coccobacillus, *Moraxella bovis*. Other agents, such as *M ovis*, *Mycoplasma boviculi*,[1,2] and *Chlamydophila* spp,[3] have been implicated. Carrier animals of *M bovis* have been identified and the spread of *M bovis* has been attributed to the face fly (*Musca autumnalis*) (**Fig. 1**).

The author has nothing to disclose.

[a] Belmont Veterinary Centre, 94 Belmont Road, Hereford HR2 7JS, England, UK

[b] Cambridge Infectious Diseases Consortium (Clinical Research Outreach Programme), Department of Veterinary Medicine, University of Cambridge, Madingley Road, Cambridge CB3 0ES, England, UK

* Belmont Veterinary Centre, 94 Belmont Road, Hereford HR2, England, UK.

E-mail address: alexanderdominic@yahoo.co.uk

Vet Clin Food Anim 26 (2010) 487–503
doi:10.1016/j.cvfa.2010.09.006
0749-0720/10/$ – see front matter © 2010 Elsevier Inc. All rights reserved.

vetfood.theclinics.com

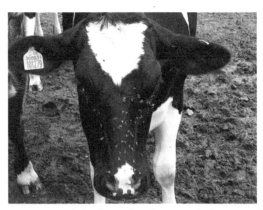

Fig. 1. Flies congregating around the face. The photograph illustrates how pathogens are transmitted.

CLINICAL SIGNS

Infectious bovine keratoconjunctivitis (IBK) is a disease principally of the cornea characterized by epiphora, lacrimation, blepharospasm, and photophobia. This can progress into corneal edema and, if left unchecked, ulceration of varying depth and diameter. Trauma, either physical or chemical, can produce clinical signs similar to IBK. Other pathogens have been implicated and can cause clinical signs that are indistinguishable from IBK.[2,4] Conjunctivitis of varying severity is sometimes seen but not in every case. This may be as a secondary consequence to the ulceration or the ulceration may arise due to the weight of infection from the inflamed conjunctiva.

During the examinations discussed in this article, it was possible to witness the initial clinical signs of an outbreak of IBK (**Figs. 2–4**).

In **Fig. 5**A, the early signs of ulceration can be seen with profuse epiphora. **Fig. 5**B exhibits similar ulceration but no epiphora. This can make early recognition and,

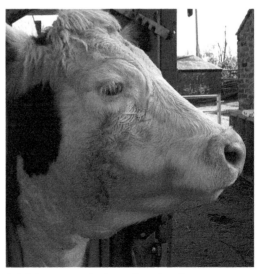

Fig. 2. Epiphora and staining are early signs of ocular disease.

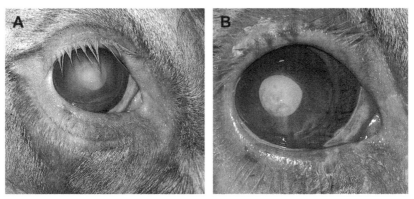

Fig. 3. (*A*, *B*) The extent of a corneal ulcer is revealed post staining with fluorescein. (*A*) Pre fluorescein staining and (*B*) post fluorescein staining.

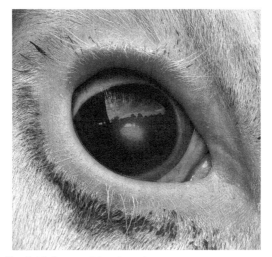

Fig. 4. The eye in **Fig. 3** 18 days post treatment.

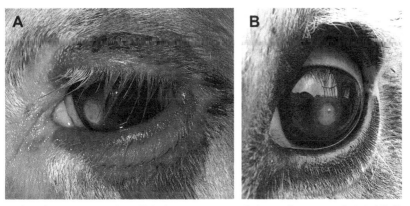

Fig. 5. (*A*, *B*) Two contrasting clinical appearances of the early stages of IBK. (*A*) Shows corneal ulceration with profuse epiphora. (*B*) Shows corneal ulceration but no corresponding epiphora.

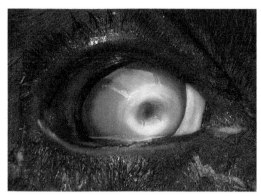

Fig. 6. A deep infected ulcer penetrating the stroma. The cornea has diffuse edema with vascularization migrating from the limbus.

hence, prompt treatment of disease difficult because severe ulceration takes hold rapidly.

Some cases of IBK spontaneously resolve. If left unchecked, however, severe damage to the cornea can arise, leading to deep ulceration and prolapse of the anterior chamber (**Fig. 6**).

Fig. 7 shows severe IBK that had not been treated, *M bovis* was cultured. The corneal ulcer had perforated with prolapse of the anterior chamber. There was no evidence, however, of prolapse of the iris.

Traumatic lesions as depicted with the laceration of the lower left eyelid of the bull in **Fig. 8** may cause either direct or indirect trauma to the cornea. The eye itself managed to escape severe damage, even perforation; however, because of the loss to the integrity of the border of the lower lid, a severe conjunctivitis ensued that began to affect the cornea.

AN OUTBREAK OF IBK IN BEEF CATTLE AT GRASS

The cases shown in this case study were animals of approximately 12 months of age grazing at grass. Approximately four adult breeding cows were also affected (**Figs. 9–12**).

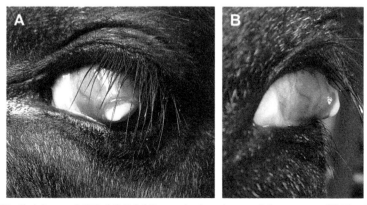

Fig. 7. (*A, B*) Advanced IBK. (*A*) Exhibits marked prolapse of the cornea. (*B*) The head-on view of the same eye seen in A illustrates the extent of the prolapse.

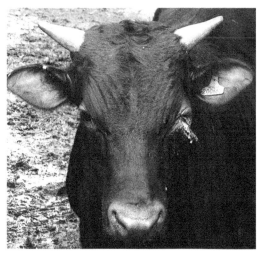

Fig. 8. A severe example of a traumatic injury that subsequently led to damage to the cornea with excessive bacterial overload.

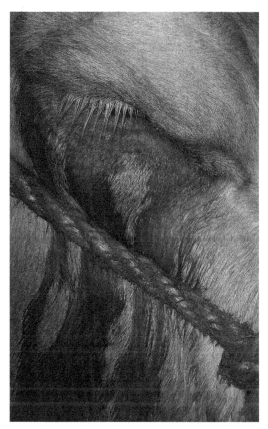

Fig. 9. Blepharospasm and lacrimation often increase as ocular disease progresses.

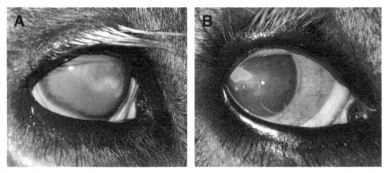

Fig. 10. (A, B) Note the blue haze—corneal edema and peripheral vascularization. The opaque area in the center of the cornea exhibits a superficial ulcer when stained with fluorescein.

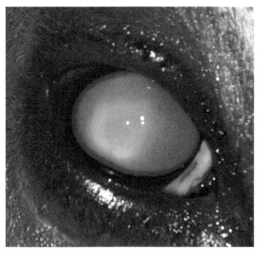

Fig. 11. The cornea showing endophthalmitis and vascularization extending from the limbus. The pupil is dilated and the IOP 44 mm Hg.

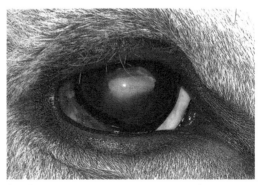

Fig. 12. Forty days after the initial examination, the cornea shown in **Fig. 11** is almost healed and the IOP down to 23 mm Hg.

A Belgium Blue cross Holstein breeding cow, approximately 5 years old, had a markedly elevated intraocular pressure (IOP) of 44 mm Hg. The unaffected left eye had an IOP of 18 mm Hg. The cow was treated with nonsteroidal anti-inflammatory drugs (NSAIDs) (meloxicam 0.5 mg per kg [2.5 ml per 100 kg]) topical and subconjunctival antibiotics. Ten days later, the pressure had reduced to 17 mm Hg in the affected right eye and was 17 mm Hg in the unaffected left eye. The elevated IOP was probably caused by inflammatory damage to the iridocorneal angle causing disruption to the flow of aqueous humor. Forty days after the initial examination, the cow eventually made a good recovery with remnants of superficial vascularization visible on the affected cornea. The IOP was 23 mm Hg in the affected right eye and 25 mm Hg in unaffected eye.

DIFFERENTIAL DIAGNOSES OF IBK AND CONCURRENT DISEASE

During an outbreak of IBK, a clinician can easily overlook other diseases. Squamous cell carcinoma is an example of a disease that can occur concurrently with IBK. Topical and systemic antimicrobial and NSAID therapy should be used followed by re-examination 5 to 7 days later (**Fig. 13**).

Removal of the affected tissue, or even enucleation, may be required if feasible. Histopathology is desirable in all suspected cases of carcinoma. The cow in the photograph (see **Fig. 13**) was treated for IBK (*Pseudomonas aeruginosa* was cultured) and the cyst on the nictitans resolved apace with the corneal ulceration.

Bovine iritis—silage eye—is a disease primarily affecting the iris. Inflammation of the iris/uveitis is the predominant feature (see article by Erdogan elsewhere in this issue). In common with IBK, however, blepharospasm, photophobia, and lacrimation are often seen together with corneal lesions (as seen in **Fig. 14**) and, thus, the conditions may be difficult to differentiate. History of big bale silage use and occurrence in winter rather than summer are differences between IBK and silage eye. Watson[5] reported an outbreak of silage eye where 50% of the cows and heifers in a dairy herd were affected over a winter period.

The eye in **Fig. 14** exhibits corneal edema, hyphema, hypopyon, and vascularization migrating from the limbus and clearly appears different from those in IBK.

The animal pictured in **Fig. 15** cultured positive for *Listeriosis monocytogenes* even though there was clear corneal ulcerative involvement. Corneal ulceration is not typical

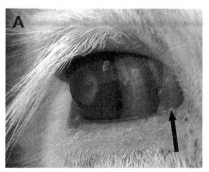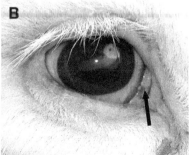

Fig. 13. (*A*) Note the small raised area/cyst (*arrow*) on the nictitans in addition to the corneal ulceration. This can be an early indication of squamous cell carcinoma. (*B*) Corneal ulceration is markedly reduced 6 days post treatment. The cyst has reduced slightly (*arrow*) and eventually disappeared.

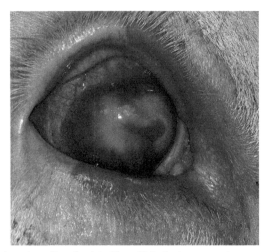

Fig. 14. Ocular lesions in a Hereford heifer—*Listeriosis monocytogenes* was identified on culture.

of silage eye; however, in clinical practice, varying degrees of corneal ulceration are often seen.

Fig. 16 depicts the clinical signs of infectious bovine rhinotracheitis (IBR) caused by bovine herpes virus 1 (BHV-1). There is a mucopurulent discharge, conjunctivitis, and congestion of the subconjunctiva. No ulceration was detected after staining with fluorescein. IBR can be diagnosed by fluorescent antibody tests in acute cases via nasopharyngeal and ocular swabs but once a mucopurulent discharge appears, secondary bacteria contaminate the swabs. Acute and convalescent serology may be the only way of historically confirming the presence of IBR.

Other diseases, such as bovine viral diarrhea virus and malignant catarrhal fever, must form part of the differential diagnosis when examining a patient. A mucopurulent discharge and conjunctivitis are often present with malignant catarrhal fever and in the acute stages of IBR. In the peracute stages of both diseases, however, mild conjunctivitis and a serous discharge may be all that are seen. The immunosuppressive affects

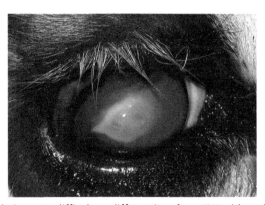

Fig. 15. Here, the lesions are difficult to differentiate from IBK, although *Listeria monocytogenes* was cultured.

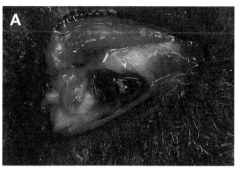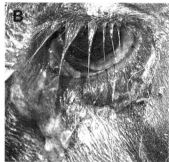

Fig. 16. (*A, B*) With IBR, severe conjunctivitis is seen with a serous discharge that became mucopurulent but without frank corneal signs.

of bovine viral diarrhea virus can readily allow ocular pathogens to manifest with greater vigor in both transiently viraemic and persistently infected animals.

Corneal and Conjunctival Cultures

Microbiologic culture swabs should be taken before putting any topical medications into the eye. Various types of swab are available, plain and those with bacterial and virus media. If there is any doubt, check with the laboratory that is testing/culturing the swabs as to what is required. Plain swabs are useful if there is uncertainty, although the pathogens are prone to desiccation. To help ameliorate dessication, dampen the swab with sterile water before taking the sample. Most samples in this study were collected and placed in tubes containing Amies transport medium with or without charcoal with a viscose-tipped polystyrene shaft. A small percentage was collected and placed in tubes without media. The pathologic samples in this article were assayed by the Veterinary Laboratories Agency (VLA).

Corneal scrapings can be useful to detect bacterial and deep fungal hyphae. Care must be taken not to cause any further damage, and topical local anesthetic (eg, proxymetacaine) must be applied before taking a corneal scraping.

Table 1 illustrates the incidence of pathogens isolates in the England and Wales. Additional laboratory testing is sometimes undertaken, either by further culture or polymerase chain reaction, to identify *Chlamydia* and *Mycoplasma* spp.

Table 2 shows the diverse range of bacteria identified. Only two pure growths of *M bovis* were cultured. This was identified from two housed, 4- month-old Belgium Blue cross Holstein heifer calves with IBK in the cold winter month of January 2010. The remaining culture was taken from a 3-year-old Holstein heifer, at grass, in mid-August 2010. Initially a mixed growth, including *Acinetobacter* species, was identified with a *Moraxella* species detected after extended culture.

The calf in **Fig. 17** was one of two calves exhibiting clinical signs that were similar to IBK: epiphora, blepharospasm, corneal edema, vascularization, and miosis of the pupil when observed with a pen torch. Both calves were male Holstein/Friesian calves of approximately 12 weeks of age. They were housed among a group of 40 similar calves. Corneal swabs were taken. Treatment immediately commenced with subconjunctival injections of oxytetracycline (100 mg/1 mL) and parenteral injections of oxytetracycline (20 mg per kg [20 mL]). Topical chlortetracycline ophthalmic ointment was applied daily and parenteral NSAIDs: initially, flunixin meglumine (2.2 mg per kg [2 mL per 45 kg]) followed by one injection of meloxicam 24 hours later (0.5 mg per kg [2.5 mL per 100 kg body weight]) (**Figs. 18** and **19**).

Table 1
The frequency of *Listeria monocytogenes* and *Moraxella bovis* identified from ocular swabs submitted to the VLA

| | Pathogens | |
Year	*Listeria monocytogenes*	*Moraxella bovis*
2001	4	10
2002	2	16
2003	4	26
2004	1	27
2005	4	8
2006	2	21
2007	3	14
2008	2	4
2009	2	18
2010	5	6

Data courtesy of the VLA.

Visible signs of healing were slow. The results from the ocular swabs were unexpected. Pure cultures of *Streptoccocus suis* were isolated from both calves. The strain of *S suis* cultured was resistant to oxytetracycline among other antimicrobials. Subcutaneous (SC) injections of tilmicosin (Micotil) (10 mg per kg [1 mL per 30 kg]) were administered to both calves and improvements could be seen within 1 to 2 days post injection.

In addition to visual examination, IOPs were taken as part of a study into bovine ocular disease. Pressures were taken with a TonoVet rebound tonometry machine.

Table 2
The type and frequency of pathogens isolated from 36 ocular swabs taken between September 10, 2009, and August 12, 2010

Pathogens Isolated	Frequency
BHV-1	2
Acinetobacter spp	2
Comamonastestosteroni and *Pseudomonas alcaligenes*	1
Heavy mixed growth of predominately *E coli*	4
Heavy mixed growth of predominately *Staphylococcus* spp	3
Listeria monocytogenes	3
Listeria monocytogenes and *Pseudomonas fluorescens*	1
Mixed growth incl *Acinetobacter* spp and *Moraxella* spp	1
Mixed flora including nonhemolytic *Staphylococcus*	1
Mixed growth	3
Moraxella bovis	2
Pantoea spp	1
Pseudomonas aeruginosa	1
Pseudomonas spp	1
Streptococcus suis	2
No growth/nothing cultured	8

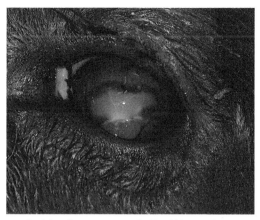

Fig. 17. IBK in a 12-week-old Holstein/Friesian bull calf housed in a straw bedded yard.

This method is less likely to cause any further damage to an already traumatized cornea. In addition, topical anesthetic, which can have deleterious affects on the restoration of corneal epithelial cells, is not required. The calves were re-examined on days 4, 7, 11, and 20 post treatment. Photographs were taken of the affected eyes along with IOPs from both the affected and unaffected eyes in both calves. Calf no. 14 had an IOP of 22 mm Hg in the unaffected left eye on the initial day of examination (day 0) and an IOP of 13 mm Hg in the affected right eye. By day 20, the corneas in both eyes had visibly begun to heal and their IOPs were of 21 mm Hg in the unaffected left eye and 17 mm Hg in the affected right eye for calf no. 14. This reduction in ocular pressure, followed by a restoration of pressure, seems to be a common feature of the convalescing eye. A small, and statistically significant, dip in pressure seems to occur in the contralateral unaffected eye. Further work is currently being undertaken in this area.

The second calf (no 15) had an IOP of 24 mm Hg in the unaffected right eye on day 0 and an IOP of 14 mm Hg in the affected left eye, again, a drop in IOP. Calf no 15 had

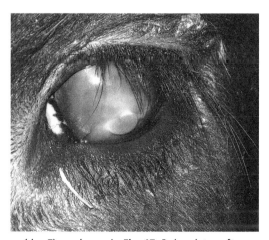

Fig. 18. The same eye (day 7), as shown in **Fig. 17**, 3 days later after a systemic injection of tilmicosin (Micotil).

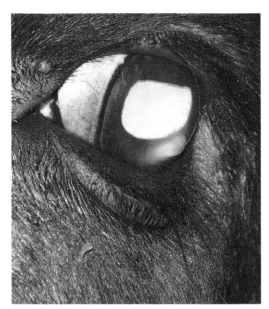

Fig. 19. Almost complete resolution by day 11.

an IOP of 25 mm Hg in the unaffected right eye and an IOP of 19 mm Hg in the affected left eye by day 20.

It will be interesting to learn, over time, whether or not IOP could be a quick and useful prognostic indicator of the health of the eye and its response to treatment.

TREATMENT OF IBK
Topical Treatment

Topical treatment can rapidly arrest the early stages of disease. The early signs, such as excess lacrimation, if noticed, usually respond rapidly to topical antibiotic treatment. The most common topical treatments used in the United Kingdom are cloxacillin and, to a lesser extent, chlortetracycline. Topical atropine (1%) drops are useful by inducing mydriasis and cycloplegia, which alleviate some of the pain of anterior uveitis by relieving ciliary body spasm. Topical atropine, however, is normally given to affect. Bovine patients are not normally readily accessible for intensive topical treatment and the mydriatic affect of atropine is extremely variable. The duration of activity can last for many days if there are no synechial attachments to impede dilation of the pupil. Therefore, the likelihood of a bovine being treated frequently is doubtful. It is worth remembering that an animal released to pasture with little shade could suffer from the affects of UV rays of bright sunlight if treated with a long-acting mydriatic, such as atropine.

Subconjunctival Treatment

Subconjunctival injections are a cost-effective way of administering antibiotics. Their use is not without controversy, in that their mode of action is debatable. There are potential risks in the administration of a depot of medication, in the bulbar subconjunctiva, in what is most probably, a fractious and painful animal. Penicillin G[6] is a universal antibiotic used for subconjunctival injection in the treatment of IBK. The recurrence of

IBK, however, in practice, seems to occur more readily with penicillin if the weight of infection is great.

It is argued that subconjunctival injections used in treating cattle are not, strictly, true subconjunctival injections in that they may be given in the upper eyelid. A subconjunctival injection should be a small depot (1 to 2 mL) of medication injected at the junction between the conjunctiva and sclera—under the bulbar conjunctiva. This technique is used in equine ophthalmology because after the initial visual and neurologic examination, patients are normally sedated. Sensory and motor nerve blocks are also performed to facilitate the safe and accurate execution of a subconjunctival injection. Many veterinarians treating an outbreak of ocular disease in cattle probably administer the antibiotic in the conjunctival tissue of the upper lid. There is much debate as to whether or not the globe receives any antibiotic at all by this method. Leakage of medication through the injection site, directly onto the cornea, however, is the most probable reason for their apparent success.

Sargison and colleagues[6] treated all 150 6-month-old calves where 85% of eyes showed signs of inflammation. The inflammation was bilateral in 75% of calves. Mixed growths of gram-negative bacilli and gram-negative cocci were cultured from conjunctival swabs at the time. *M bovis*, *M branhamella ovis*, *Neisseria* spp, and *Staphylococcus* spp were identified. Isolation of *M bovis* from conjunctival swabs collected 9 days post treatment indicated either failure to eliminate the pathogens or re-infection. The merits of whole-group treatment were not elucidated because it was not possible to establish how bad the outbreak would have been if the entire group had not been treated. In New Zealand, where this study was undertaken, farmers believe that IBK is a self-limiting disease and, in many incidences, does not warrant treatment. The welfare implications of such an approach are debatable.

Oxytetracycline is often the second treatment of choice after penicillin. Oxytetracycline seems to be irritant[7] to the tissues of the upper eyelid and increased swelling is a consequence. This, nevertheless, may limit the ability of the animal to open the upper eyelid giving added protection to the cornea in a manner similar to temporary tarsorrhaphy, where the eyelids, or the third eyelid (nictitans), are temporarily sutured. In New Zealand, farmers sometimes glue some stiff paper to the area above the upper eyelid (over the orbital fossa and caudal edge of the temporal process). This is said to improve rates of recovery probably by providing protection from UV light (sunlight) in a manner similar to the peak of a baseball cap.

A trial undertaken by Senturk and colleagues[8] used clindamycin as the antimicrobial for subconjunctival injection. The study used 46 animals with naturally occurring IBK, ie, the animals were not experimentally inoculated with *M bovis*. The results were encouraging with good cure rates along with no recurrence noted within the 15 days' monitoring period post treatment. Clindamycin is not licensed for use in food-producing animals in the United Kingdom so its use in clinical practice cannot be validated.

Fluoroquinolones should not be used as a first-line of treatment. In some countries, including the United States, their use in food animal medicine is not permitted. Due to a large outbreak of IBK that was slow to respond to topical treatment with either chlortetracycline or cloxacillin and subconjunctival injections of oxytetracycline or penicillin, respectively, marbofloxacin (1 to 2 mL [10–20 mg]) was given as a subconjunctival injection. Response to therapy was good; however, it seemed to cause the patients some discomfort as it was injected, probably more than oxytetracycline, which is tolerated less well than penicillin G. During this outbreak, heavy mixed and pure growths of *E coli* and *Staphylococcus* were cultured, which explains the pure initial response to treatment. Kibar and colleagues[9] reported using the fluoroquinolone, enrofloxacin, as a subconjunctival to successfully treat a herd outbreak of IBK.

Florfenicol is a derivative of chloremphenicol. It has been used by the authors as a subconjunctival injection on a few occasions. It seemed to be successful in the treatment of IBK. The solution is viscous, however, and difficult to inject. Angelos and colleagues[10] found that it was successful in treating IBK when given systemically. The use of florfenicol is discussed later.

Atropine has been given as a bulbar subconjunctival injection in conjunction with dexamethasone by the authors in severe cases of miosis. Approximately 2 mg of atropine and 2 mg of dexamethasone are given by injection. Good physical restraint, chemical sedation, and often an auricular palpebral nerve block are required to enable the medication to be given safely. Bulbar subconjunctival injection of dexamethasone and atropine is a procedure that is only undertaken on a few animals.

Systemic Treatment

Systemic treatments can be an attractive alternative to subconjunctival injections. Their significant advantage is that less restraint is required to administer the medication, which is safer for both patients and clinicians. Systemic treatment involves antibiotics and NSAIDs that are probably underused. Systemic treatment is more expensive due to the quantity of drug used. Speed and safety of administration, however, along with longevity/duration[7] of therapy are superior to topical and subconjunctival therapy.

Several antimicrobials are used: oxytetracycline, florfenicol, tilmicosin, and ceftiofur. Systemic treatment is not a common mode of treatment in the United Kingdom. Cost, ease of administration, and milk and meat withdrawal periods are important considerations. Judicious and sensible use of antibiotics should be at the forefront of a clinician's mind. Antimicrobial resistance is not normally a major deliberation when deciding on a treatment regime but, increasingly, it should be.

Most antibiotics are licensed to treat four major ailments that affect cattle: bovine respiratory disease, mastitis, uterine infections (metritis and endometritis), and lameness due to infections of the lower limb (eg, foul in the foot). Ocular disease represents only a small amount of disease treated by farmers or veterinarians. It is not cost effective for pharmaceutical companies to license their products for the treatment of bovine ocular disease; moreover, attempts to ascertain the clinical effectiveness of the various methods of delivering the drug would be very laborious, time-consuming and extremely expensive (eg, subconjunctival vs systemic and the various routes by which systemic treatment can be delivered).

Tulathromycin (Draxxin) is a semisynthetic macrolide antimicrobial that is licensed for treating pneumonia in cattle and IBK. Its use in the United Kingdom has increased due to the changes to the licensing of tilmicosin (Micotil), which can now only be administered by veterinarians. After a single SC administration (2.5 mg/kg), tulathromycin reaches a peak plasma concentration of 414 ng/mL by 0.25 hours.[11] Lane and colleagues[11] state that a strain of M bovis (Tifton-1) was susceptible to concentrations of tulathromycin greater than 0.5 μg/mL which is an easily achievable concentration in parentally treated calves. Tulathromycin is low dose and has prolonged activity. It does, however, have a long meat withdrawal period of 49 days in the United Kingdom and is not licensed for use in animals producing milk for human consumption. It could prove a useful and cost-effective treatment for young calves and significantly reduce the risk of re-infection.

Ceftiofur crystalline-free acid (CCFA) was assessed by Dueger and colleagues.[12] It is the free acid form of ceftiofur held in a sterile vegetable oil suspension. Ceftiofur is a broad-spectrum, β-lactamase–resistant, bactericidal cephalosporin and was developed as a single-dose treatment for respiratory disease in cattle. It now has a zero milk withhold license for use in lactating cattle for the treatment of acute interdigital necro-bacillosis, associated with *Fusobacterium necrophorum* and *Bacteroides melaninoge-nicus*. It has a license for use in the treatment of metritis in some countries. The drug is administered by SC injection at the base of the ear. Dueger and colleagues[12] cite a 4 to 5 fold increase in the odds of a corneal ulcer attributed to *M bovis* healing by day 14.

CCFA has only recently been licensed in the United Kingdom. The authors have wit-nessed encouraging results in IBK, where mixed bacterial infections have been signif-icantly difficult to clear. Administration of the drug has been easy when the animal has been adequately restrained. Little resistance or movement was observed and the systemic administration of medication, in this manner, is easier and less stressful for patients and clinicians. The risk of further ocular trauma while trying to administer SC medication is alleviated and a low-dose volume is convenient when treating several animals in a herd outbreak. A 400-kg animal requires 13.3 mL CCFA. A zero milk withhold for milk-producing animals and a 9-day meat withdrawal facilitates treat-ing cattle nearing slaughter.

Florfenicol is an effective treatment for IBK.[10,13] A study was undertaken by Angelos and colleagues[10] where it was administered at the concentration advocated for treat-ment of bovine respiratory disease. It was given either as a single SC dose (40 mg/kg) or two intramuscular injections (20 mg/kg, 48 hours apart). Its down side is its high-dose volume. A 400-kg animal requires approximately 53 mL as a single SC dose. Newer formulations are more concentrated and less viscous. Nonetheless, a 400-kg animal still requires 35 mL SC. This can make the physical task of administering the medication strenuous and time consuming in a large outbreak. Gokce and colleagues found that healing times were shorter in calves treated with florfenicol than in calves treated with oxytetracycline. Two groups of 15 calves were given either florfenicol or oxytetracycline in two intramuscular injections (20 mg/kg, 48 hours apart). Relapse was not observed in calves treated with florfenicol compared with those treated with oxytetracycline.[13]

MEAT AND MILK WITHHOLD TIMES

When treating clinical cases of IBK, it is important to be aware of the withhold times. A study by Liljebjelke and colleagues[14] found that penicillin G could be detected in milk up to 22 hours post–bulbar subconjunctival administration of only 300 mg/1 mL (300,000 units) of penicillin. In the United Kingdom, for example, some preparations of procaine benzylpenicillin have a milk withhold of between 3.5 days (84 hours) and 11 days (204 hours) at a dose rate of 12 mg per kg body weight. This means that although only small amounts of antibiotic are used in subconjunctival injections, full withdrawal periods should be adhered to. The use of ceftiofur sodium, ceftiofur hydro-chloride, and CCFA may be of great benefit to milk producers in countries/provinces where these cephalosporin compounds have a milk withdrawal time of zero hours.

WELFARE IMPLICATIONS

Several of the figures in this article illustrate the huge welfare implications of IBK, with severe ulceration occurring and also often secondary uveitis. (Welfare implications are discussed elsewhere in this issue in the article by Williams.) Prompt topical treatment often prevents the disease progressing any further. When stock are at pasture, careful examination is difficult. NSAIDs could significantly reduce intraocular inflammation and pain, but their use is often precluded by economic and management issues.

PREVENTION

M bovis is ever-present. More often than not it does not lead to clinical disease. Because the majority of diagnosis is made on clinical signs alone, how can the clinical disease of IBK be prevented if the organism is not necessarily going to be *M bovis*? Spread between animals can be reduced by the use of fly repellents/insecticides (eg, deltamethrin). This has been the authors' experience until a recent herd outbreak of IBK where *M bovis* was not isolated. Although heavy pure and mixed growths of *E coli* and *Staphylococcus* were identified, spread of infection throughout the herd did not seem to reduce postapplication of insecticide. Direct contact should be minimal because the cattle were at pasture and not receiving supplementary feed, which can allow increased head-to-head contact at the feed trough.

VACCINATION

No vaccines against *M bovis* are currently available in the United Kingdom. In light of the mixed infections identified, it is debatable how a nonmultivalent vaccine could be efficacious. Davidson and Stokka[15] were not able to show any statistical difference between vaccinated and unvaccinated calves. George and colleagues,[16] however, illustrated some resistance to *M bovis* post inoculation with a cytolysin-enriched vaccine devived from a hemolytic strain of *M bovis*.

The overall results on vaccination of the calves infection and disease were considered ambiguous. Pugh and colleagues[17] noticed specific results from different selection lines indicated that vaccination reduced the carrier status for up to 9 months, which also caused a reduction in the percentages of calves with IBK in three of the four of these selection lines.

MANAGEMENT

Active cases of IBK attract flies. Lacrimation and staining of the face attract flies. The flies pick up *M bovis* and pass it on to a neighboring animal where they too may succumb to IBK. Reducing exposure to flies, by removing cattle from wooded areas or standing water, is often impractical. Moreover, although fires may be more prevalent in wooded areas, trees do provide shade, which can help to reduce the deleterious affects of UV light.

A severe outbreak occurred in some housed Holstein heifers of approximately 12 months of age. They were treated with subconjunctival penicillin G and topical cloxacillin. The heifers began to recover but would then relapse. As fast as one heifer was treated, another began to show clinical signs. Although housed, a huge number of flies were noted in the open-sided building. Their origin seemed to be from a large mound of decaying apple pumice tipped in a silage clamp close to the building. Application of an insecticide, deltamethrin, plus removal of the apple pumice halted the incidence of IBK virtually overnight. It would have been interesting to have trapped some flies and seen if they were carrying *M bovis* but unfortunately none were caught. Removal of their breeding ground, however, and the use of a fly repellent had such a dramatic result that the farmer became convinced of preventative measures where he had not appreciated their benefits before.

SUMMARY

In conclusion, IBK is a complicated multifaceted disease. It is often said that prevention is better than cure, and this is nowhere more appropriate than in IBK. Preventative measures need to be improved and hard work is needed to ascertain the most efficacious treatments through rigorous evidence-based medicine.

REFERENCES

1. Angelos JA, Spinks PQ, Ball LM, et al. Moraxella bovoculi sp. nov., isolated from calves with infectious bovine keratoconjunctivitis. Int J Syst Evol Microbiol 2007; 57:789–95.
2. Angelos JA. Moraxella bovoculi and infectious bovine keratoconjunctivitis: cause or coincidence? Vet Clin North Am Food Anim Pract 2010;26:73–8.
3. Otter A, Twomey DF, Rowe NS, et al. Suspected chlamydial keratoconjunctivitis in British cattle. Vet Rec 2003;152:787–8.
4. Levisohn S, Garazi S, Gerchman I, et al. Diagnosis of a mixed mycoplasma infection associated with a severe outbreak of bovine pinkeye in young calves. J Vet Diagn Invest 2004;16:579–81.
5. Watson CL. Eye disease in the growing animal—can we prevent it? Cattle Pract 2006;12:213–8.
6. Sargison ND, Hunter JE, West DM, et al. Observations on the efficacy of mass treatment by subconjunctival penicillin injection for the control of an outbreak of infectious bovine keratoconjunctivitis. N Z Vet J 1996;44:142–6.
7. Brown MH, Brightman AH, Fenwick BW, et al. Infectious bovine keratoconjunctivitis: a review. J Vet Intern Med 1998;12:259–66.
8. Senturk S, Cetin C, Temizel M, et al. Evaluation of the clinical efficacy of subconjunctival injection of clindamycin in the treatment of naturally occurring infectious bovine keratoconjunctivitis. Vet Ophthalmol 2007;10:186–9.
9. Kibar M, Gumussoy KS, Ozterk A. Evaluation of various antibiotic treatments in calves with infectious bovine keratoconjunctivitis. Turk J Vet Anim Sci 2006;30:553–9.
10. Angelos JA, Dueger EL, George LW, et al. Efficacy of florfenicol for treatment of naturally occurring infectious bovine keratoconjunctivitis. J Am Vet Med Assoc 2000;216:62–4.
11. Lane VM, George LW, Cleaver DM. Efficacy of tulathromycin for treatment of cattle with acute ocular Moraxella bovis infections. J Am Vet Med Assoc 2006; 229:557–61.
12. Dueger EL, George LW, Angelos JA, et al. Efficacy of a long-acting formulation of ceftiofur crystalline-free acid for the treatment of naturally occurring infectious bovine keratoconjunctivitis. Am J Vet Res 2004;65:1185–8.
13. Gokce HI, Citil M, Gerc O, et al. A comparison of the efficacy of florfenicol and oxytetracycline in the treatment of naturally occurring infectious bovine keratitis. Ir Vet J 2002;55:573–6.
14. Liljebjelke KA, Warnick LD, Witt MF. Antibiotic residues in milk following bulbar subconjunctival injection of procaine penicillin G in dairy cows. J Am Vet Med Assoc 2000;217:369–71.
15. Davidson HJ, Stokka GL. A field trial of autogenous Moraxella bovis bacterin administered through either subcutaneous or subconjunctival injection on the development of keratoconjunctivitis in a beef herd. Can Vet J 2003;44:577–80.
16. George LW, Borrowman AJ, Angelos JA. Effectiveness of a cytolysin-enriched vaccine for protection of cattle against infectious bovine keratoconjunctivitis. Am J Vet Res 2005;66:136–42.
17. Pugh GW Jr, McDonald TJ, Kopecky KE, et al. Infectious bovine keratoconjunctivitis: comparison of infection, signs of disease and weight gain in vaccinated versus non-vaccinated purebred Hereford heifer calves. Can J Vet Res 1986;50:259–64.

Listerial Keratoconjunctivitis and Uveitis (Silage Eye)

Hidayet Metin Erdogan, DVM, PhD

KEYWORDS

- Cattle • Listeria • Keratoconjunctivitis • Uveitis • Silage eye
- Silage feeding

Listeriosis is a bacterial zoonotic disease caused by the genus *Listeria*, especially *Listeria monocytogenes*.[1–4] The disease is manifested by 3 distinct clinical patterns, which are encephalitis, abortion, and septicemia in both humans and animals.[5,6] In addition, mastitis,[7] iritis, and/or keratoconjunctivitis[6,8–15] have also been associated with *L monocytogenes* infection in ruminants in recent years.

Listeria has attracted considerable attention owing not only to increased reports of clinical disease in animals[2,6,16] and people[3] but also to its implication as a foodborne pathogen.[1,4]

ETIOLOGY

The origin of keratoconjunctivitis comprises many infectious agents, including *L monocytogenes*.[15,17] Listerial keratoconjunctivitis or silage eye is always associated with *L monocytogenes* and silage feeding.[2,10,11,14,15,18]

L monocytogenes is a gram-positive, non–spore-forming, noncapsular, short, regular rod. Listerial organisms can multiply from around 0°C to around 50°C, with optimal growth being between 30°C and 37°C.[19,20] *L monocytogenes* can also tolerate a wide range of pH (3.8–9.2).[21] The tolerance to this broad range of temperatures and pH enables *L monocytogenes* to survive and grow indefinitely in the environment. *Listeria* spp are aerobic or facultatively anaerobic organisms.[2] In anaerobic conditions, *L monocytogenes* cannot survive at a pH of less than 3.8,[18,22] but exposure to oxygen makes it possible for *L monocytogenes* to survive even if the pH is as low as 3.8.[18] Therefore, anaerobic conservation of silage is important, as silage has long been associated with *L monocytogenes* infection and is thought to be the source of the organism.[2,5,16,20,22]

Division of Veterinary Clinical Science, Department of Internal Diseases, Faculty of Veterinary Medicine, University of Kafkas, 36100 Kars, Turkey
E-mail address: hmerdogan@hotmail.com

Vet Clin Food Anim 26 (2010) 505–510
doi:10.1016/j.cvfa.2010.09.003
0749-0720/10/$ – see front matter © 2010 Elsevier Inc. All rights reserved.

PATHOGENESIS

The ways in which *L monocytogenes* reaches and causes systemic illness have long been the subject of interest. The existence of different forms of clinical listeriosis and their irregular distribution in animals suggest that *L monocytogenes* gains entry in several ways.[2] The pathogenesis is thus poorly defined.[23]

Experimental and clinical cases disclosed the main portal of entry as the oral route, bruised mucosa (oral or conjunctival), inhalation, and direct or indirect contact with contaminated materials.[23,24] Studies have supported the hypothesis that *L monocytogenes*–contaminated forages, such as grass, silage, grain awns, straw, and hay, can break up the integrity of the mucosal membranes and allow *L monocytogenes* to penetrate.[2,24]

Erdogan[2] found a strong association between silage eye and the use of big bale silage and silage feeding in ring feeders, as it is already reported that animals eating silage in ring feeders and from big bales were at a greater risk of exposure to the agent and physically damaging their conjunctival membranes,[2,9,14,15,18,25] because there is a continuous exposure of the eye to silage in such feeding methods, which may lead to infection of epithelial cells of the cornea and conjunctiva by *L monocytogenes*,[26] resulting in eye inflammation. Although listerial keratoconjunctivitis has long been reported, the pathogenesis of the disease remains to be fully described.[15]

EPIDEMIOLOGY

Keratoconjunctivitis is a widespread disease of the ruminants, causing distress to animals and economic losses to farmers. The epidemiology of listeriosis has extensively been studied in general, but the epidemiology of listerial keratoconjunctivitis has not yet been studied in detail. The disease has been reported from different parts of the world, especially Europe and the United Kingdom, where silage feeding is a common practice.[6,8–15]

Outbreaks of listerial keratoconjunctivitis have occasionally been reported.[8–15] The morbidity rate may vary between 25% and 100%,[18] the farm prevalence was 8.6%, and the incidence rate in all herds and affected herds were reported as 3.4% and 66.5%, respectively, by Erdogan and colleagues.[6] Erdogan[2] also reported that the most common clinical sign was the silage eye (83.7%) and that most cases occurred in late autumn, winter, and spring when animals were housed and silage feeding was exercised.

Silage and farm environment are thought to be the sources of the infection, as contamination of the agricultural ecosystem with *L monocytogenes* is well documented and *L monocytogenes* is thought to be a saprophytic organism living in a plant-soil environment. Carrier humans and animals are thought to play an essential role in the contamination of their environment (eg, vegetation, soil, water).[2,27–32]

Listerial keratoconjunctivitis has always been related to silage feeding.[14,18] This suggestion was supported by the findings of a PhD study performed by Erdogan.[2] In that study, unconditional logistic regression analyses of survey data revealed a significant relationship between silage and the disease. Use of big bale silage, silage feeding in ring feeders during the indoor period, ad libitum silage feeding from clamp during the outdoor period, improper silage making (soil contamination), unsuitable housing conditions (overcrowding), and presence of other animals with clinical listeriosis on the farm significantly increased the risk of listerial keratoconjunctivitis.[2] In addition, other factors that may increase the susceptibility of animals to listeriosis, possibly to listerial keratoconjunctivitis as well, include poor nutritional state, sudden changes to very cold and wet weather, stress of late pregnancy and parturition, and overcrowded and unsanitary conditions with poor access to feed supplies and poor herd or flock management.[33,34]

Clinical Signs

The disease is named as listerial keratoconjunctivitis,[15] iritis,[10,35] uveitis,[18,36] silage eye,[6,25] and ophthalmitis.[37] Lesions are located unilaterally or bilaterally, but most lesions are unilateral. Morgan[9] reported 2 outbreaks of the disease; the lesions were a catarrhal conjunctivitis with epiphora and photophobia, moderate ophthalmitis with hydrophthalmus and hypopyon, and keratitis in the first outbreak and severe ophthalmitis with marked hydrophthalmus, hypopyon and iridocyclitis, and conjunctivitis and moderate involvement of the cornea in the second. The course of the disease was about 7 to 10 days in these outbreaks, and no residual lesions were reported. Staric and colleagues[15] reported keratoconjunctivitis manifested by excessive lacrimation, blepharospasm, photophobia, blindness, yellowish anterior chamber fluid and corneal opacity of varying degree, turbidity of anterior chamber, anterior uveitis, and hyperemic conjunctiva. Keratitis manifested by punctate abscesses, peripheral clouding, and epiphora and iritis have also been associated with *L monocytoegens* infection in cattle.[12] Uveitis/anterior uveitis or iritis was reported in deer, sheep, and cattle.[10,11,14,18,25,35–37] Sargison[18] described the signs of uveitis as excessive lacrimation, blepharospasm, photophobia, miosis, and iridocyclitis followed by swelling and undulating folds in the iris and ciliary body; severe inflammatory changes with bluish white corneal opacity starting at the limbic border and spreading centripetally within 2 to 3 days; accumulation of focal aggregation of fibrin in the anterior chamber attached to the inner surface of the cornea; accumulation of white material beneath the cornea, hypopyon, and mild conjunctivitis at the period of inflammation; pannus with widespread corneal opacity; and vascularizations spreading from the limbus in more severe cases. The course was reported to be 1 to 3 weeks if not treated.[18] Similar clinical signs and inflammatory changes in the eyes of cattle and sheep were also reported by other researchers.[10–12,35,36,38]

Listerial keratoconjunctivitis and uveitis have been reported as primary conditions, which are not associated with other clinical signs of listeriosis.[10,14,15,18] No report of nervous listeriosis following anterior uveitis exists except for that of Ohshima and colleagues,[38] in which cerebral listeriosis was reported to be present along with uveitis.

Diagnosis

Clinical signs involving the uvea are typical, and history of silage feeding may help in diagnosis, but the exact diagnosis is based on the demonstration of *L monocytogenes* from the samples collected from the affected eye. Conventional or molecular techniques (eg, polymerase chain reaction) are sufficient to detect *Listeria* in affected materials.[2]

Differential diagnosis of listerial keratoconjunctivitis may include infectious bovine keratoconjunctivitis (IBK) associated with *Moraxella bovis* and other agents. Uveal changes make the disease distinct from IBK because IBK produces severe conjunctivitis, lacrimation, blepharospasm, photophobia, intense corneal changes, and corneal ulceration in more severe cases and occurs most commonly in summer and autumn when flies are active.[9,18,34,35]

Treatment

Treatment of listerial keratoconjunctivitis includes parenteral and/or topical use of antibiotics. Morgan[9] reported the use of chloramphenicol powder with less effect. Sargison[18] and Blowey[35] reported the success of the subconjunctival use of the combination of oxytetracycline and dexamethasone. Walker and Morgan[37] used topical oxytetracycline in sheep but found it ineffective; they then administered parenteral ampicillin plus topical ceprovin, which led to the recovery of cases within 2 weeks. Mee and Rea[36] also reported the recovery of cows with uveitis within 2 weeks of administration of systemic antibiotics and antibiotic-corticosteroid ophthalmic ointment, although they did not mention the names of the drugs used. Evans and colleagues[12] reported the recovery of 3 cases after the use of topical antibiotic ointment in one case, atropine and oxytetracycline plus polymyxin B sulfate ophthalmic ointment in the second case, and subcutaneous injection of procaine penicillin G in the third case. Staric and colleagues[15] also reported complete healing after systemic and topical antibiotic use but did not mention the name of the antibiotics used. Reports revealed that systemic or topical use of antibiotics or a combination of both with or without corticosteroid resulted in complete recovery within 2 weeks in almost all cases. Recovery without any treatment was also reported.[9,12]

Control

Because the elimination of *L monocytogenes* from the farm environment is not possible because of its ubiquitous occurrence in nature, the lack of reliable and rapid methods of detecting the organism when it is present in low numbers, and the lack of understanding of the epidemiology of listeriosis and *L monocytogenes* infection, attempts can be made only to prevent listerial organisms from multiplying to the level of an infectious dose, minimize its presence in the farm environment by improving hygiene and cleanliness of the farm, and minimize its intake by animals by preparing foodstuff such that *L monocytogenes* does not grow.[2] The most important risk factor of listerial keratoconjunctivitis is silage feeding, as all clinical cases were linked to silage feeding, especially big bale silage, and problems ceased after removing silage from the diet.[2,9,15] Wherever silage is implicated, some recommendations can be made. The proportion of silage in the ration can be reduced, silage feeding can be introduced to the animals gradually, and more attention can be paid to silage making. Spoiled and moldy silage should be removed from the feed. When making silage, additives should be used, soil contamination should be avoided, and the silo or clamp should be sealed off as quickly as possible so that an anaerobic condition is maintained and the pH is kept low.[2,34,39] The method of silage feeding should be changed so that eye contact can be minimized, that is, not using ring feeders, direct feeding from clamps, and big bale silage.[2] Better farm management practices, such as the improvement of nutritional status of animals, better housing conditions, and good hygiene and cleanliness, can also be of some value in preventing the disease.[2,34]

REFERENCES

1. Farber JM, Peterkin PI. *Listeria monocytogenes*, a foodborne pathogen. Microbiol Rev 1991;55:476–511.
2. Erdogan HM. An epidemiological study of listeriosis in dairy cattle [PhD thesis]. United Kingdom: University of Bristol; 1998.
3. Lecuit M. Human listeriosis and animal models. Microbes Infect 2007;9:1216–25.
4. Ramaswamy V, Cresence VM, Rejitha JS, et al. Listeria–review of epidemiology and pathogenesis. J Microbiol Immunol Infect 2007;40:4–13.
5. Gray ML, Killinger AH. *Listeria monocytogenes* and listeric infections. Bacteriol Rev 1966;30:309–82.

6. Erdogan HM, Cetinkaya B, Green LE, et al. Prevalence, incidence, signs and treatment of clinical listeriosis in dairy cattle in England. Vet Rec 2001;149: 289–93.

7. Gitter M, Bradley R, Blampied PH. *Listeria monocytogenes* infection in bovine mastitis. Vet Rec 1980;107:390–3.

8. Kummeneje K, Mikkelsen T. Isolation of *Listeria monocytogenes* type 04 from cases of keratoconjunctivitis in cattle and sheep. Nord Vet Med 1975;27: 144–9.

9. Morgan JH. Infectious keratoconjunctivitis in cattle associated with *Listeria monocytogenes*. Vet Rec 1977;100:113–4.

10. Watson CL. Bovine iritis [letter]. Vet Rec 1989;124:411.

11. Bee DJ. Ovine iritis [letter]. Vet Rec 1993;132:200.

12. Evans K, Smith M, McDonough P, et al. Eye infections due to *Listeria monocytogenes* in three cows and one horse. J Vet Diagn Invest 2004;16:464–9.

13. Akerstedt J, Hofshagen M. Bacteriological investigation of infectious keratoconjunctivitis in Norwegian sheep. Acta Vet Scand 2004;45:19–26.

14. Laven RA, Lawrence KR. An outbreak of iritis and uveitis in dairy cattle at pasture associated with the supplementary feeding of baleage. N Z Vet J 2006;54:151–2.

15. Staric J, Krizanec F, Zadnik T. *Listeria monocytogenes* keratoconjunctivitis and uveitis in dairy cattle. Bull Vet Inst Pulawy 2008;52:351–5.

16. Gitter M. Veterinary aspects of listeriosis. PHLS Microbioliology Digest 1989;6: 38–42.

17. Baptista PJ. Infectious bovine keratoconjunctivitis: a review. Br Vet J 1979;135: 225–42.

18. Sargison N. Health hazard associated with the feeding of big bale silage. In Pract 1993;2:291–7.

19. Juntilla JR, Neimele SI, Hirn J. Minimum growth temperature of *Listeria monocytogenes* and non-haemolytic *Listeria*. J Appl Bacteriol 1988;65:321–7.

20. Erdogan HM, Cripps PJ, Morgan KL. Optimisation of a culture technique for the isolation of *Listeria monocytogenes* from faecal samples. J Vet Med B Infect Dis Vet Public Health 2002;49:502–6.

21. Picard-Bonnaud F, Cottin J, Carbonnelle B. Persistence of *Listeria monocytogenes* in 3 sorts of soil. Acta Microbiol Hung 1989;36:263–7.

22. Fenlon DR. Growth of naturally occurring *Listeria* spp. in silage: a comparative study of laboratory and farm ensiled grass. Grass and Forage Science 1986; 41:375–8.

23. Vázquez-Boland J, Kuhn M, Berche P, et al. *Listeria* pathogenesis and molecular virulence determinants. Clin Microbiol Rev 2001;14:584–640.

24. Asahi O, Hosoda T, Akuyama Y. Studies on the mechanism of infection of the brain with *Listeria monocytogenes*. Am J Vet Res 1957;18:147–57.

25. Welchman DD, Hooton JK, Low JC. Ocular disease associated with silage feeding and *Listeria monocytogenes* in fallow deer. Vet Rec 1997;140:684–5.

26. Zimianski MC, Dawson CR, Togni B. Epithelial cell phagocytosis of *Listeria monocytogenes* in the conjunctiva. Invest Ophthalmol 1974;13:623–6.

27. Weis J, Seeliger HP. Incidence of *Listeria monocytogenes* in nature. Appl Microbiol 1975;30:29–32.

28. Watkins J, Sleath KP. Isolation and enumeration of *Listeria monocytogenes* from sewage, sewage sludge and river water. J Appl Bacteriol 1981;50:1–9.

29. van Renterghem B, Huysman F, Rygole R, et al. Detection and prevalence of *Listeria monocytogenes* in the agricultural ecosystem. J Appl Bacteriol 1991;71:211–7.

30. Nightingale KK, Schukken YH, Nightingale CR, et al. Ecology and transmission of *Listeria monocytogenes* infecting ruminants and in the farm environment. Appl Environ Microbiol 2004;70:4458–67.

31. Ivanek R, Grohn YT, Wiedmann M. *Listeria monocytogenes* in multiple habitats and host populations: review of available data for mathematical modeling. Foodborne Pathog Dis 2006;3:319–36.

32. Mohammed HO, Atwill E, Dunbar L, et al. The risk of *Listeria monocytogenes* infection in beef cattle operations. J Appl Microbiol 2010;108:349–56.

33. Hyslop NStG. Epidemiologic and immunologic factors in listeriosis. In: Woodbine M, editor. Proceeding of the 6th international symposium on the problems of listeriosis. England, Nottingham (UK): Leicester University Press; 1975. p. 94–105.

34. Radostits OM, Blood DC, Gay CC. Veterinary medicine. London. 8th edition. Philadelphia: Bailliare Tindall; 1994. p. 660–6.

35. Blowey RW. Ovine iritis. Vet Rec 1993;132:444.

36. Mee JF, Rea M. Baled silage associated with uveitis in cows [letter]. Vet Rec 1989;124:25.

37. Walker JK, Morgan JH. Ovine ophthalmitis associated with *Listeria monocytogenes*. Vet Rec 1993;132:636.

38. Ohshima K, Mira S, Mumakunai S, et al. Case of bovine cerebral listeriosis with ocular lesions. Jap J Vet Sci 1974;36:183–5.

39. Fenlon DR. Listeriosis. In: Stark BA, Wilkinson JM, editors. Silage and health. Aberystwyth (UK): Chalcombe Publications; 1988. p. 7–19.

Bovine Ocular Squamous Cell Carcinoma

Hiroki Tsujita, DVM, Caryn E. Plummer, DVM*

KEYWORDS

• Bovine • Squamous cell carcinoma • Eye • Ocular neoplasia

Ocular squamous cell carcinoma (OSCC) in animals is a primary neoplasm of epithelial origin that may occur in different ocular and periocular tissues, especially the epithelial surfaces of conjunctiva, corneoscleral junction, nictitating membrane, and cornea and the eyelid skin. OSCC is a spontaneous tumor, which occurs with high frequency globally in bovines.

OSCC or "cancer eye" is the most common malignant tumor affecting cattle in North America and is responsible for significant economic losses.[1–5] The occurrence of OSCC has been reported worldwide, in Europe, Asia, Africa, Australia, and South America.[6–10] In Australia, 10% to 20% of animals in some herds have been diagnosed with OSCC.[11] In Zimbabwe, European breeds of cattle and their crosses, particularly those with unpigmented skin on the face, are commonly observed to have OSCC.[12] The incidence of OSCC in the United Kingdom and other European countries is lower than in Africa and the Americas; however, it is still a significant disease.[6,13,14] In the Netherlands, the incidence is 0.04% based on examination of 35,000 animals.[15] OSCC is found primarily in cattle, although it has been observed at a low incidence in sheep, swine, goats, and horses.[16]

In the United States, the prevalence of OSCC varies with geography and is higher in the southwestern region and in lower latitudes with higher levels of sunlight.[14,17,18] This pattern is similar to that observed with human skin-cancer cases.[4] Lightly pigmented human skin when chronically exposed to sunlight may undergo a series of changes, commencing with the development of keratoses and frequently progressing to basal cell opthollomas or squamous cell carcinomas (SCCs). There have been some studies on the spontaneous development of similar lesions in animals exposed to intense sunlight.[4,19,20] Some breeds of cattle, especially the Hereford, are noted for their high incidence of carcinomas when kept in subtropical areas. Sheep develop

Departments of Small and Large Animal Sciences, Comparative Ophthalmology Service, University of Florida, College of Veterinary Medicine, PO Box 100126 Gainesville, FL 32610-0126, USA
* Corresponding author.
E-mail address: PlummerC@ufl.edu

Vet Clin Food Anim 26 (2010) 511–529
doi:10.1016/j.cvfa.2010.08.003
0749-0720/10/$ – see front matter © 2010 Elsevier Inc. All rights reserved.

vetfood.theclinics.com

carcinomas, apparently associated with exposure to sunlight, on areas of the integument unprotected by fleece, particularly the ears, muzzle, and perineal area.[20]

OSCC is the leading cause of whole-carcass condemnation at slaughter. The disease comprises 80% of all bovine tumors reported at slaughter.[14] High morbidity rates of 0.2% to 5.6% result in significant economic loss from culling and condemnation.[3,4,21,22] Control of this disease would be of considerable significance to the economics and profitability of the beef and dairy cattle industries.

Although a common tumor, the genesis of OSCC has not been fully investigated, and several theories have been advanced to explain its development, including breed susceptibility, influence of exposure to ultraviolet (UV) light, viral infection, age and gender, and nutritive conditions. Various treatment options for OSCC exist: surgery, cryosurgery, radiation therapy, immunotherapy, and hyperthermia have been recommended in many studies. This article reviews the characteristics of the most commonly affected animals, the factors that are believed to contribute to the development of OSCC and the treatment options that have been proposed.

ETIOLOGY

The cause of OSCC is still poorly understood; however, there are several factors including genetic susceptibility, nutrition levels, age, UV light, circumocular apigmentation, and viruses that may contribute to its development.

Breed Susceptibility

Cases of OSCC have been reported in Holstein-Friesian, Holstein, Hereford, Guernsey, Shorthorn, Ayrshire, Brahman, Brown Swiss, Hollandensa, Javanese-Mongolian, Jersey, and Normandy breeds of cattle, among others.[13,14,23] Although it has been reported in many different breeds, this invasive, chronically progressive neoplasm predominantly affects Hereford, Hereford cross, and Holstein cattle. At the University of Florida, the frequency of OSCC is particularly high in the white-faced Hereford. This breed is commonly kept in an environment favorable for the development of OSCC and has a hereditary inclination towards facial hypopigmentation. Holsteins with pink skin around the eyes are more susceptible to OSCC (**Fig. 1**).

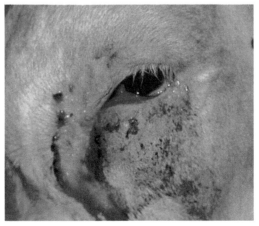

Fig. 1. SCC lesion involving the lower eyelid, nictitating membrane, and conjunctiva in a Holstein cow with pink skin.

The Hereford breed in the United States has an estimated incidence of 0.8% to 5% of this disease compared to 0.8% to 1.6% in the general cattle population.[24,25] Anderson[18] presented data on nearly 1500 cattle of 6 different breeds and various Hereford crosses. Of 696 purebred Herefords in this group, 25.3% had cancer eye or early lesions suggestive of OSCC. Only 17.7% of 261 Hereford crosses and one Holstein out of 140 were observed with the disease. In this study, no tumors were found in Angus, Shorthorn, Santa Gertrudis, or Scottish Highland cattle (see **Fig. 1**).

Genetic factors other than hypopigmentation of the periocular tissues are also likely to be involved. Several investigators have studied the influence of heredity.[22,25] Historical investigations have studied the progeny of animals with and without OSCC, and the incidence of disease is greater in animals born to affected animals.

Blackwell and colleagues[26] investigated the inheritance of susceptibility with data from 415 of 630 animals, from 209 dams and 31 sires. Of 350 matings in which neither parent was affected, only 11% of the progeny developed OSCC. Of 140 matings in which only the sire or the dam had cancer eye, the incidence among progeny was 26% and 22%, respectively. These results suggest that inheritance is an important factor in the occurrence of OSCC, with approximately 20% to 30% of the total variability due to additive effects of genes. Genetic studies in OSCC have been carried out to evaluate 2 major aspects of inheritance: the inheritance of susceptibility independent of environment factors and the genetic relationship between eye pigmentation and OSCC.[4]

Sites of Predilection

Most studies to date have reported on the relationship between environmental levels of UV light and epithelial pigmentation when discussing predilection sites. Lack of circumocular pigmentation is thought to play a major role in the susceptibility, induction, and promotion of the carcinogenesis of OSCC, because melanin plays a photoprotective role in epidermal and mucosal surfaces. In a survey of 842 mature cattle, 17.6% with no lid pigmentation in either eye had tumor lesions.[27] In another study of tumors that have developed in partially pigmented eyelids, the investigators have concluded that lesions develop primarily in the unpigmented areas.[10,28] Similarly, Stewart and colleagues[12] reported that OSCC in Zimbabwean cattle are frequently observed in European breeds of cattle and their crosses that have unpigmented periocular skin. Often, these animals have been kept at high altitude and exposed to intense solar radiation for long periods.[29] Hereford and Hereford crosses commonly have white faces and periocular hypopigmentation; this undoubtedly contributes to the high incidence of disease in this breed.

The most common sites of OSCC development are the lateral conjunctiva and corneolimbal junction (**Figs. 2, 3** and **4**). The lower eyelid (**Fig. 5**A, B), nictitating membrane (**Fig. 6**A, B, C), and medial canthus are less commonly affected sites. Conjunctival SCC is well described in cattle, and the lesions most commonly occur along the line of palpebral closure, most often on the lateral rather than the medial conjunctiva.[14] The nictitating membrane has been postulated to have an important role in protecting the medial conjunctiva from exposure to UV radiation and the irritative effect of foreign bodies, thus reducing the incidence of conjunctival SCC in the medial half of the bulbar conjunctiva.[14]

UV Light

UV radiation is thought to be related to the initiation of SCCs in cattle, horses, and cats.[30] There is strong evidence that in cows, the prevalence of SCC is related to sunlight overexposure.[5] The affected animals tend to be kept at high altitude and/or

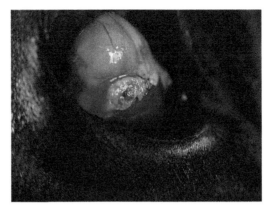

Fig. 2. Bovine limbal SCC. The most common sites of OSCC development are the lateral conjunctiva and corneolimbal junction. (*Courtesy of* Dr Murakami, DVM, Nakasorachi AMAA, Hokkaido, Japan.)

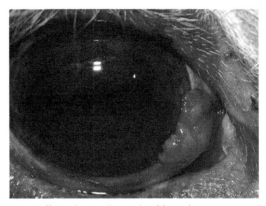

Fig. 3. Limbal squamous cell carcinoma in a mixed-breed cow.

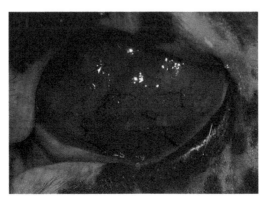

Fig. 4. Corneal SCC.

exposed to intense solar radiation for long periods of time. In humans, exposure to excessive UV light has been identified by numerous studies as a major etiologic risk factor in the development of ocular surface squamous neoplasia.[31] SCC of the conjunctiva undoubtedly has a multifactorial cause, but exposure to solar UV radiation is considered a major contributor to its development. UV radiation is thought to cause DNA damage and the formation of pyrimidine dimers. Failure or delay in DNA repair may lead to somatic mutations and the development of cancerous cells, as occurs in human patients with xeroderma pigmentosa.

In recent years, many studies have suggested that mutations of the p53 tumor suppressor gene are involved in the development of human sunlight-related skin cancers, namely SCC and basal cell carcinoma, and of UV-induced SCC of mice.[32]

This gene encodes for a 53-kDa nuclear phosphoprotein, which functions as a regulator of cellular growth and proliferation, and it functions in the control of the cell cycle, of DNA repair, and of the apoptotic pathway. UV radiation is known to arrest some cells during the G1 phase of the cell cycle in a p53-dependent manner. Once DNA is damaged, the nuclear p53 protein concentration sharply rises because of a post-translational stabilization mechanism.

Using immunohistochemical techniques, Carvalho and colleagues[1] investigated whether the degree of differentiation of OSCC could be correlated with p53 overexpression and with proliferative activity of tumor cells. OSCC samples were collected from 15 bovines, and 10 of 15 tumors tested were immunoreactive for p53. In this study, high levels of labeling were obtained with antihuman p53 CM-1 polyclonal antibody in 67% of the OSCCs. In all cases that tested positive, p53 immunoreactivity was restricted to the nuclei of tumor cells. These data indicate that p53 accumulation in the nucleus of cells is common in OSCC. In another study, Teifke and Lohr[30] analyzed skin SCCs immunohistochemically for overexpression of p53 protein in 106 SCCs of cattle, horses, cats, and dogs. OSCCs in bovines showed 63.4% p53 nuclear reactivity. All equine OSCC gave positive reactions. In 81.8% of feline SCC of the ear and 50% of feline SCC of other locations, p53 immunoreactivity was detected. Only 29.5% of canine cutaneous SCC gave a positive reaction. Cells testing positive were observed predominantly in the periphery of the typical "pearls" of SCC but not in their keratinized centers. Atypical cells with a high nucleus/cytoplasm ratio showed a strong immunoreactivity against mutant p53 in most cases. In these reports, it was shown that immunoreactivity for mutant p53 occurs frequently in different SCCs of the skin, and the results of this investigation support the view that, as in the human, p53 overexpression plays an important role in the development of most SCCs of the animal species studied and that UV radiation may be the initial cause of most SCCs.

Viruses

A viral cause has been suspected for many years, and several independent studies have demonstrated viruses or viruslike particles in tumor tissue.[9,33–36] Many possibilities exist as to the role such herpes viruses and/or papillomaviruses may play in the sequential development of benign precursors and their progression to SCC.

Taylor and Hanks[36] collected biopsy samples from 32 bovine eyes in a Nevada abattoir. In this study, infectious bovine rhinotracheitis (IBR) was isolated from the carcinomas collected. The tumors used in the study included corneal OSCC in early and late stages, as well as tumors excised from nictitating membranes. Correlations of serum neutralizing titers against IBR in normal cattle and in cattle affected with eye tumors were also reported in this study. In the normal group, serum neutralizing antibody titers for IBR were detected in the sera of 29% of 96 animals tested. In the group affected with OSCC, serum neutralizing titers were observed in 84% of 19

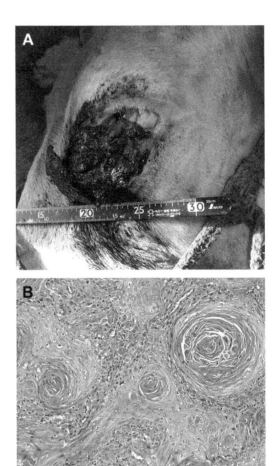

Fig. 5. (*A*) Extensive, ulcerated SCC in situ of the medial aspect of the lower eyelid in a Holstein cow. (*Courtesy of* Dr Sato, DVM, Azabu University, Kanagawa, Japan.) (*B*) The tumor is composed of islands and trabeculae of neoplastic epithelial cells, showing varying degree of squamous differentiation. Central accumulation of dense laminated keratin (keratin pearls) are present in variable size and numbers. (*Courtesy of* Dr Kondo, DVM, University of Florida, Gainesville, FL, USA.)

animals tested. These results supported earlier observations of *herpes-type* inclusion bodies reported in histologic studies of OSCC lesions. Collectively, the presence of intranuclear inclusion bodies in cancer eye lesions, the isolation of herpes viruses from OSCC, the fact that herpes viruses induce tumors in their natural hosts, the ability of UV light to induce herpes viruses to transform cells, and the presence of several types of herpes virus that infect cattle suggested that a herpes virus may be involved in the cause of OSCC.

However, Anson and colleagues[37] reported that virus was not isolated from tissue homogenates of 31 bovine ocular tumors processed in their study. They concluded that previous isolation of IBR by other groups was simply of passenger viruses, because most herpes viral tumors yield infectious virus only after induction by UV light, steroids, or pH changes. However, they were able to demonstrate tumor cell-associated antigens that reacted to herpes virus 5 (DN-599) antisera by indirect immunofluorescence

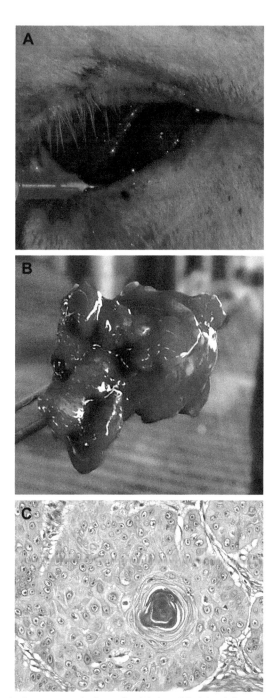

Fig. 6. (*A*) Neoplastic tissue protrudes from the third eyelid of the right eye of a Holstein cow. (*B*) Histologically, the lesion was a squamous carcinoma. (*C*) Histopathologic findings. The neoplastic cells have abundant eosinophilic cytoplasm and round-to-ovoid nuclei with stippled chromatin and 1 to 2 large nucleoli. There are individual dyskeratotic cells. Intercellular bridges are obviously observed. (*Courtesy of* Dr Kondo, DVM, University of Florida, Gainesville, FL, USA.)

on tumor cells grown in cell culture. UV light, 5-Iodo-2'- deoxyuridine, and high pH media were used to induce virus replication in tumor cell cultures, and the number of tumor cells expressing bovine herpes virus 5 antigens increased after exposure to UV light or maintenance in media at pH 8.4. The ability of UV light to induce viral antigens in vitro is interesting, because prolonged exposure of cattle to UV or sunlight increases the incidence of OSCC. These results suggest that BHV-5 may be associated with OSCC, and further studies are required to substantiate this theory.

Viruses other than herpes have been implicated in the development of OSCC, especially the papillomaviruses. The bovine papillomavirus (BPV) has been suggested to be involved in the development of bovine OSCC, especially in precursor lesions of OSCC.[33,34,36,37] BPV has also been proposed as a causative agent associated with equine sarcoid and bovine skin papilloma.[19,31,38] Bovine and ovine carcinomas develop from wartlike precursor lesions, which have been shown to contain papillomaviruses.[34] Ford and colleagues[34] suggested that infection with papillomavirus and exposure to sunlight, possibly together with other factors, such as a period of photosensitization, are involved in the production of this spectrum of proliferative lesions, which bear some resemblance to human skin cancer. The alteration of the microenvironment with respect to cell-cell and/or cell matrix interactions on the limbus, the area of transition from conjunctival to corneal epithelium, may result in an altered regulatory mechanism of the limbal stem cell function, leading to abnormal epithelial phenotypes. OSCC may represent the abnormal maturation of corneal and conjunctival epithelium as a result of a combination of factors, such as UV-B irradiation and BPV. A recent review, however, using DNA probes and electron microscopy, failed to detect the direct involvement of BPV DNA.[31] It was concluded that BPV may contribute to induction of precursor lesions or events leading to carcinogenic transformation, without being relevant to the maintenance of the tumor.

Age

The peak incidence of OSCC in the bovine occurs between 7 and 8 years of age, although animals younger than 3 years have been reported, rarely, with OSCC.[29] A study of disposal records of cattle over a 21-year period reported that the rate of culling seems to increase linearly with age until a peak age of incidence between 7 and 9 years.[18] In this study, a very high incidence in animals of 12 to 14 years of age was reported, but few animals this advanced in age were present in the herds. The low population of old animals may artifactually skew the study results; however, a continued increase in the cumulative percentage incidence may indicate that when animals are retained in the herd to older ages, the incidence of cancer eye is likely to increase. Den Otter and colleagues[29] also described that in some herds, more than half of the older cattle may be affected. Other studies have also reported an increasing prevalence of this condition with increasing age.[14,18,21,39] Although the age pattern may reflect only the consequences of prolonged exposure to carcinogens, it may also indicate biochemical or immunological alterations that increase with age. The phenomenon of cancer in older animals is probably due to prolonged exposure, which increases the chance over time that the interaction of multiple factors results in tumorigenesis.

Gender

It is not known whether the sex of the animal is an important factor in this disease.

However, as for horn SCC in cattle, Dugan and colleagues[41] and Lall[42] proposed that sexually intact male and female cattle are significantly less likely to develop horn SCC than castrated male cattle, because of increased circulating androgens and estrogens.[40–42] The difference in these hormones between castrated and sexually intact animals may provide an explanation for the increased frequency of OSCC and adnexal SCC in geldings.

Wernicke[43] considered the disease to be more common in the female sex than the male, but this finding was intuitive, because 9 of the 12 diseased animals included in his pedigree were female and only 3 were male. On the other hand, Blackwell and colleagues[26] concluded that no apparent sex difference in incidence of cancer eye was found in this study. Of 40 male animals with records available, 4 developed cancer eye. The expected number, if the incidence was the same as among female cattle, was 5. There is no scientific data to suggest that the female is more susceptible to OSCC than the male of the same age. However, cows may be more commonly affected simply because of the female sex predominance in older cattle populations, not necessarily because of a predilection of OSCC for the female sex. For economic reasons, most cases are naturally among cows, because steers are sent to slaughter, whereas young and mature cows are kept for breeding and stay in the herd as long as they remain productive and healthy.

Nutritive Conditions

It has been suggested that high levels of nutrition were correlated with an increased incidence of OSCC. A study by Anderson[18] reported that cattle maintained on a minimal nutrition level had a lower rate of OSCC.[18,44] Those maintained on high levels had a higher incidence of tumors and a greater number of affected sites per animal, higher incidences at younger ages, and more progressive disease. These findings indicate a possible physiologic effect of high levels of nutrition on tumor development. Further study is necessary to substantiate and investigate this possibility.

CLINICAL FINDINGS AND DIAGNOSIS

Bovine OSCCs can occur at different sites on the eye. Common sites for OSCC include the lower lid, the third eyelid, and the corneoscleral junction of the globe. Both eyes are often affected to a varying degree.

OSCC often exhibits benign precursor lesions, referred to as plaques, although no apparent de novo appearance of malignant lesions has been observed. Generally, the disease progresses through 3 defined stages: plaques, papillomas, and carcinoma. Typically, the carcinoma arises from plaque and papilloma precursor lesions on and around the epithelial tissue of the periocular and ocular structures. These lesions occur most commonly at the corneoscleral junction and on the lower eyelid. Cordy[45] reported that the most common site (75%) is the limbus or the junction of the cornea and the sclera, and the eyelids, including the third eyelid account for the other 25%. Similarly, Farris and Fraunfelder[46] showed the distribution of locations for OSCC to be most common on the limbus (43%) in 295 cattle, with a total of 609 OSCC lesions. Thirty-five percent were on the eyelid, 12% were seen on nictitating membrane, and 10% were on inner canthus. These distributions are different from the findings of some authors.[12,47] In the study by Stewart and colleagues[12] of the 174 tumors, 37% cases were on the third eyelid; 25%, the limbus; 23·5%, the lower eyelid; 14%, the canthus; and one tumor involved the whole eye. Stewart described 3 possible reasons for the differences. First, only tumors more than 1 cm in diameter were included, and the small plaques that frequently occur on the limbus and often regress by themselves were therefore not included. Second, this study dealt with live cattle, whereas some of the other studies dealt with slaughtered animals examined at abattoirs, from which third eyelid tumors may have been removed. Third, it is possible that OSCCs may have different predilection sites for Zimbabwean cattle as a result of genetic differences or different causes.

There are 4 stages in the development of OSCC. The first is a plaque (stage 1), followed by keratoma or keratoacanthomas (stage 2), papillomas (stage 3), and finally, carcinomas (stage 4). The initial plaques appear as small, raised, white areas in the affected tissue. Keratomas occur more frequently on the lower eyelid and are skin growths coated with eye secretions and debris.[12] Papillomas may have a wartlike, proliferative appearance, and carcinomas are more irregular and nodular and may be pink from an increased vascular supply. Plaques, keratomas, and papillomas (stages 1, 2 and 3) are benign, although as precursor lesions, they can progress to carcinomas. Without treatment, OSCC may metastasize to the regional lymph nodes and lungs. Although most lesions occur at the limbus and small benign precursor lesions often regress, tumors of the lower lid and nictitating membrane pose a greater threat, because they tend to be aggressive and are more likely to metastasize. Carcinomas (stage 4) are malignant, and all tumors more than 2 cm in diameter are, by definition, carcinomatous.

Diagnosis of OSCC is usually made by the typical clinical appearance, but can be confirmed rapidly by cytologic examination of impression smears or histopathologic examination of biopsy specimens. Pretreatment diagnostic techniques, such as impression cytology, are of great value and can aid clinical decision-making and the follow-up management; however, cytology should not be used as an alternative to histopathology. Severe inflammatory reactions may cause a false diagnosis of OSCC, and the cytologic findings should be compared with histopathologic findings.

Histologically, OSCC may range from well-differentiated to undifferentiated anaplastic carcinoma. The histology of early lesions demonstrates a bandlike mononuclear cell infiltrate in the upper dermis. Even early lesions may show considerable hyperplasia and dysplasia of the epithelial layer. More advanced lesions show invasion of the subepithelial tissues, further dysplastic or anaplastic changes to the epithelial cells, formation of keratin pearls, and evidence of vascular or lymphatic spread.

The likelihood of metastasis of OSCC varies with the location of the primary tumor. Tumors in the eyelids show a higher frequency of metastases than tumors of the cornea and limbus; Hamir and Parry[3] reported that metastases were seen in 11% of cows suffering from invasive carcinoma of the eye or eyelids, and Russell and colleagues,[14] in 1% of cows suffering from OSCC of the eyelids. In both studies, the presence or absence of lung metastases was not reported. Another study reported that 61% of 21 animals with an enlarged subparotid lymph node had regional lymph node metastases and 6 of these animals also had lung metastasis.[15]

TREATMENT OF OSCC

Many therapeutic protocols have been described for OSCC in different primary sites, and they have varying levels of difficulty, required equipment, and results.[12,15,41,46–55] Previously described options include surgical excision, cryotherapy, radiofrequency hyperthermia, immunotherapy, chemotherapy, and radiation therapy.

Surgical Excision

Excision of the lesions is the most accepted method of treatment for squamous neoplasia of the ocular surface (bulbar conjunctiva, corneolimbal and corneal tissue). Dissection of all abnormal tissue within a wide surgical margin of 2 to 3 mm around the periphery of the lesions is usually sufficient to ensure removal of most lesions. A superficial keratectomy, wherein the epithelial and anterior stromal surfaces of the affected tissue are removed, is the surgical approach. Bovine limbal OSCC cases should not be treated with surgical excision alone. Additional forms of therapy, including cryotherapy, hyperthermia, and radiation therapy, are necessary to destroy the remaining tumor cells that may be present in the deeper stroma.[40,46–52]

Lesions of the eyelid are harder to completely excise. Surgical procedures for small eyelid lesions include excision alone and excision with minor reconstruction. The prognosis with this conservative surgery is considered good, and a low recurrence rate has been shown.[12,15,48] For advanced lesions of the eyelid, however, more radical surgical techniques have been used.[15] Enucleation has been generally recommended for these situations, with a favorable prognosis if the operation is performed early and if it involves complete removal of all neoplastic tissue. Simple excision of larger lesions does not suffice, because the defect created in the eyelid results in functional impairment, threatens the protection and integrity of the globe, and usually has a poor cosmetic result. Large ($\geq$50-mm diameter), locally infiltrative tumors of the lower eyelid tend to be minimally responsive to cryotherapy, hyperthermia, and immunotherapy alone; therefore, radical excision is necessary.[12,15,49–52,56]

For the eyelid-mass removal surgery, retrobulbar and modified Peterson eye blocks worked equally well in providing anesthesia to the region.[15,48] Sensation of the lower eyelid arises from the ophthalmic, maxillary, and mandibular branches of the trigeminal nerve, which emerge from the foramen orbitorotundum within the orbit and exit along the lower bony rim to innervate the skin of the lower lid. If desensitization of the lower eyelid is inadequate after retrobulbar or modified Peterson blocks or if desensitization of the lower eyelid alone is desired, infiltration of a local anesthetic along the bony rim in a line block may be performed. Akinesia of the eyelids, which facilitates surgery in the standing animal, is accomplished by selectively desensitizing the auriculopalpebral nerve.

Several techniques for resection with reconstruction have been described, and the choice of which is most appropriate for any given lesion depends on the lesion's size and location (upper or lower eyelid, medial or lateral canthus) and the amount of adjacent skin that is available for reconstruction.[12,15,48,56] The sliding skin graft, also called an h-plasty is the most commonly used technique. In this procedure, the lesion is excised and tissue from the leading margin of the wound edge is freed from its underlying attachments and advanced into the defect resultant from the excision. If possible, the nasolacrimal puncta should be preserved to maintain tear drainage; the lower fornix should be preserved because of its role in tear dynamics; and the edge of the grafted skin should be lined on its bulbar aspect with conjunctiva or similar replacement tissue. Certainly, if this is not possible without leaving affected or suspicious tissue, these aspects of lid function should be sacrificed. However, if so much tissue is removed that the lids do not adequately protect the globe, enucleation or exenteration should be performed instead. H-plasty may be considered for large infiltrative masses on the lower lid 50 mm in diameter or larger, with deep infiltration of the lid but without evidence of bony involvement or metastasis or involvement of both puncta at the medial canthus. Other skin releasing techniques, such as the Z-plasty, may facilitate skin movement for large tumors that extend an excessive distance from the lid margin. If large infiltrative tumors of the lower lid are untreated or inappropriately treated, the lid may be destroyed. Loss of the ventral cul-de-sac formed by the lower lid and conjunctiva that funnels tears toward the puncta for drainage results in epiphora, which creates a favorable environment for flies and bacteria.

Cure rates with surgical excision as high as 90% have been reported,[56] but the recurrence rate can be as high as 45%.[57] In animals without enlargement of subparotid and/or retropharyngeal lymph nodes, local surgery is sufficient in most cases, although a 37% recurrence rate has been observed after local surgery.[15] This 37% recurrence rate is similar to the 48% reported by Kleinschuster and colleagues,[58] but is much higher than the 2.5% reported by Theilen and Medwell,[59] combining local surgery with local irradiation with strontium 90 (Sr90). From a practical point of view, local surgery is the method of choice in animals without lymph node enlargement, although one should be guarded about overall prognosis. For animals with an easily palpable lymph node, radiographic examination of the lungs is indicated, to look for evidence of further metastasis.

Cryotherapy

Cryotherapy for OSCC is a relatively simple and rapid procedure that treats OSCC by causing tumor cell death and necrosis via freeze-thaw damage.[46,51] It is generally effective and relatively inexpensive. Additionally, cryosurgery provides analgesia for several months because of sensory nerve injury. This procedure causes minimal side effects and may be repeated. Cryotherapy seems to be effective because malignant cells are more sensitive to the effects of cryodestruction than normal cells.

Most often, cryotherapy is used after surgical debulking. However, it can be used as solo therapy with very small or early lesions. Cryosurgery involves the controlled application of a cryogen to tissue that the surgeon wishes to destroy. The equipment is easy to operate, and the procedure is markedly safer than irradiation options. Liquid nitrogen, the coldest cryogen at −196°C, seems to be the most popular agent, especially for treating superficial tumors, and because OSCC begins as a superficial tumor, it is amenable to this freezing technique. Liquid nitrogen can be applied by various methods. An open spray or closed-tipped probe are used to treat the affected tissue in 2 successive applications, also called double freeze-thaw technique. An open-spray type is most common. This method is most effective and allows coverage of the entire surface of a larger lesion in just a few seconds. A closed-tipped cryosurgery method, however, provides a more controlled freeze than open spray. Studies have shown efficacy or cure rates ranging from 60% to 90% with cryotherapy of not-yet invasive lesions. Cryotherapy is not recommended for tumors larger than 50 mm in diameter or for those in which the margins are ill-defined. Massive tissue necrosis with loss of the eyelid can be seen if lesions are too large for this type of therapy.

Farris and Fraunfelder[46] reported about 718 OSCCs in cattle treated with various cryosurgical units and techniques. In this study, in 609 of the lesions, a single freeze was used, with a cure rate (total regression) of 66%. In 109 lesions treated with a double freeze-thaw cycle (rapid freeze to −25°C and unaided thaw followed immediately by refreezing to −25°C), the cure rate was 97%. The most important factor in the success or failure of cryotherapy is the degree and depth of freezing. It has been shown that cryodestruction of neoplastic tissue occurs most readily when the tissue temperature is rapidly reduced to –20°C, followed by a slow, unassisted thaw. Withrow[60] reported that theoretically, the −20°C lethal zone of the ice ball is the central 75% of the ice ball, and this zone extends to a depth of about one–third of its diameter. There is also a definite relationship of tumor size and margin definition to the success of therapy. In the same study by Farris and Fraunfelder,[46] eyelid lesions treated with cryotherapy had a higher cure rate (complete regression in 75%) than lesions of the corneoscleral junction (complete regression in 59%). This may be because it is not possible to put thermocouple needles in the globe to determine tissue temperatures. Instead, corneoscleral lesions are frozen until a grossly visible ice ball extends 0.3 to 0.5 mm beyond the tumor margins.

Within one to 2 hours of the cryosurgical insult, considerable edema develops in the surrounding normal tissue because of vasculature damage. The lesion appears dark and hemorrhagic because of stagnation and diapedesis of red blood cells. During the next few days, the edema subsides, and the destroyed tissue begins to shrink and become somewhat dry. The destroyed tissue usually sloughs off in 7 to 10 days, but occasionally, it remains in place, somewhat like a bandage. Scar formation is minimal and white hairs grow around the edge of the scar. In cattle, the complications of cryosurgery are relatively few. Loss of hair in the treated area is usually transitory, secondary infections are extremely rare, and intraocular hemorrhages are only occasionally observed.

Hyperthermia

Hyperthermia is also a fairly effective and easily applied treatment modality for OSCC. Hyperthermia has been induced in neoplastic tissues by immersion of affected parts in hot water (44.5°C–48°C) for varying lengths of time in humans, dogs, rabbits, and mice.[61–63] In cattle, tumors have been heated by localized electric current fields.[49,50] A handheld radiofrequency device capable of heating ocular tumors in cattle is available and has been used for electrothermally induced regression of OSCC in cattle.[48,50] The device can induce a temperature of 50°C at a depth of 3 to 4mm over an area of 1 cm^2.[62] For cancer cells and normal cells, there seems to be a logarithmic linear relationship of cell death to temperature and time. Thus, temperature and duration of treatment are very important. Grier and colleagues[49] and Kainer and colleagues[50] reported that 50°C for 30 s/cm^2 is sufficient to kill eyelid OSCC in cattle and horses with this radiofrequency localized current field device.[49,50] In this study, 60 of 76 tumors regressed completely after a single treatment. After a second treatment, 9 tumors among the remaining 16 also regressed completely. Overall, 90.8% of the tumors regressed completely.

Grier and colleagues[49] indicated that bovine corneal SCC can be heat-treated with appropriate techniques without serious injury to normal tissue. However, if surface applications overlap from opposite directions, corneal perforation may occur. This is extremely important, considering that the bovine cornea is 0.75- to 0.85-mm thick at the corneoscleral junction. Topical anesthesia and adequate head restraint are prerequisites for preventing physical disruption of the tumor and unnecessary exposure of normal cornea to electrodes. Tumors larger than 50 mm in diameter and those with deep eyelid involvement or conjunctival penetration do not respond well to hyperthermia. The best responses of OSCC to hyperthermic therapy were in tumors less than 25 mm in diameter.[41,49,50]

Immunotherapy and Chemotherapy

Methods of enhancing an individual's immune system to induce tumor regression have been used since the nineteenth century. Several variations of immunotherapy have been used for the treatment of OSCC, including tumor-derived vaccines, nonspecific immunogens, and cytokine therapy.[11,12,29,47,53–55,58,59,64–76]

Spradbrow and colleagues[11] successfully induced tumors to regress by a single intramuscular injection of the aqueous phase of a saline-phenol extract prepared from OSCC collected from cattle. This tumor regression was associated with a cell-mediated immune reaction. After a single intramuscular injection of a saline phenol extract of OSCC, regression and sometimes complete disappearance of the tumor occurred in 85% of treated animals, and even tumors as large as 50 mm in diameter regressed completely. These findings have been confirmed by other groups of researchers.[64,65]

Peri- or intratumoral injections of bacillus Calmette-Guérin (BCG) has also been used to induce tumor regression.[47,58,65–68] This product is a cell wall extract from mycobacteria that has been used for immunotherapy for various tumors in cattle and horses and is also used as a vaccine against tuberculosis. Its use may result in complete tumor regression in 60% to 70% of animals after a single intralesional injection. However, in 50% of these animals, the tumor recurred locally, and only 30% to 40% remained tumor-free. In a study that compared this treatment option with radical surgery, the surgical cases fared better with a cure in 90% of animals.[15] A regression rate of 88% for tumors less than 25 mm in diameter, 70% for tumors 25 to 70 mm, and 0% for tumors larger than 70 mm has been reported for intralesional injections of BCG cell wall or live vaccine.[69] Some tumors as large as 50 mm in diameter showed evidence of complete regression, but the best results occurred in tumors that were 25 mm or smaller.[68] Multiple or repeated intralesional injections may have better regression rates and tumor-free intervals and lower incidences of recurrence. The use of intralesional immunogens, such as saline-phenol tumor extract and BCG, is limited to eyelid lesions and should not be used for corneolimbal or conjunctival lesions.

Several trials in human patients with cancer,[70] veterinary patients with cancer,[71,72] and mice[72,73] have shown that combining interleukin (IL)-2 with other traditional cancer therapies has resulted in excellent responses to therapy. IL-2 has innate effects on tissues, such as stimulation of neutrophils and macrophages and vascular damage resulting in leakage, in addition to its immunostimulating effects of antigen presentation and T-cell proliferation. It mediates the immune system through T-helper cell 1 skewing.[74] Local IL-2 injection therapy can be preferable to standard treatments, such as surgery, because it can be used to treat large numbers of animals in a short space of time, especially since slow-release forms of IL-2 have been developed. Studies of European breeds of cattle with OSCC in Zimbabwe and the Netherlands showed that treatment with 10 injections containing 200 000 IU IL-2 gives good therapeutic results (67% complete remissions after 20 months) without noticeable side effects and little, if any, post-treatment scarring of the delicate periocular tissue.[75,76] Rutten and colleagues[76] successfully treated OSCC in 5 cows by local treatment with IL-2. Other studies in cattle, other animals, and human beings have shown that the peri- or intratumoral infiltration of low doses of IL-2 is far more successful than high systemic doses.[12,29,53] Local IL-2 therapy causes minimal side effects, with some local swelling and edema at the tumor site but no adverse systemic effects. In contrast, when Rosenberg and colleagues[77] used high systemic doses of IL-2 combined with systemic infusions of lymphokine-activated killer cells for the treatment of human patients with cancer, there were high levels of adverse side effects, and in only about 10% did the tumor regress completely.

The efficacy of IL- 2 therapy was confirmed in a study by Stewart and colleagues.[12] One hundred seventy-four tumors of different sizes in cattle were treated daily with injections of 1 ml of solvent, or 1 ml containing 5000, 20,000, 200,000, 500,000, 1 million, or 2 million U of IL-2 for 10 days, injected as close to the base of the tumor as possible. The results indicate that low peritumoral doses of IL-2 were useful in the treatment of the tumors, and there were no significant differences between the growth rates of the tumors treated with different doses. The doses between 5000 and 200,000 U produced excellent responses at 9 months, but these responses were not maintained. The responses at 9 months to the doses between 500,000 and 2 million U were not as great, but these responses were maintained or improved with no further growth between 9 and 20 months. There was a difference in the relative growth and response to treatment of the tumors dependent on their position, a new finding in this study. The clinical responses of the treated limbal and third eyelid tumors were significantly different ($P<.05$) from the responses of the control group and the treated canthus and lower eyelid tumors. There was no significant difference between the responses of the controls and the treated canthus and lower eyelid tumors. Third eyelid tumors seem to be more sensitive to IL-2 therapy than the tumors found at other periocular sites.

Radiation

Radiation therapy has also been reported to be effective treatment for OSCC.[65,78] Generally, irradiation alone is not recommended; it is used usually as an adjunctive treatment for diffuse or spreading lesions or for pretreating to shrink lesions that are too large to be excised primarily. Previous studies indicate that ocular and adnexal SCCs treated with adjuvant radiation therapy have a lower recurrence rate than those treated without adjuvant radiation therapy, especially in lesions affecting the third eyelid.[40,79]

Options for radiation therapy include Sr90, cobalt 60 (Co60), gold 198, iridium 192 (Ir192), cesium 137, iodine 125, radon 222, and implantation of isotopes that emit gamma radiation.[40] Sr90 is a beta source that delivers 100% of its dose in the most superficial layers of the tumor location. Sr90 is successful for corneolimbal lesions after surgical debulking, and it can be easily applied after keratectomy. Complications with use of Sr90 include telangiectasia of the conjunctiva, punctate corneal ulceration, corneal edema, corneal neovascularization and scarring, iris atrophy, symblepharon, and ptosis.[40,80–84] Sr90 is only indicated for superficial tumors that are or have been debulked to a tumor depth 3 mm or less, because 80% of the radiation dose is absorbed in the first 2 mm of tumor.[40,85] A more appropriate treatment for tumors larger than 3 mm is Ir192 interstitial implants that have a radiation penetration depth of approximately 1 to 1.5 cm. Because of the delivery mechanism, this treatment is most often used for eyelid and periocular tumors and should not be considered for tumors on the globe.[86–88] Co60 teletherapy has a large penetration depth and is used for more invasive tumors, particularly as a palliative therapy.[88] Radiation therapy is one of the most effective therapies for deeply infiltrative cases; however, it can be costly and its availability is limited, particularly in light of potential personnel hazards.

SUMMARY

Of the production animal species, cattle are most affected by ocular and periocular neoplasia. OSCC is the most common neoplasia among them. In 2002, OSCC was the third-leading cause of carcass condemnation at US Department of Agriculture-Inspected slaughterhouses.[48] OSCC is estimated to cause annual losses of $20 million in the United States alone.[48] Further studies are necessary to further identify and detail the etiologic factors that contribute to the development of bovine OSCC, so that more precise recommendations for therapy and preventative strategies may be established. At present, the best outcomes are seen with small lesions treated early. Diligent monitoring for the presence and progression of lesions as well as proper husbandry and early intervention is critical to reducing or controlling the morbidity of the disease.

REFERENCES

1. Carvalho T, Vala H, Pinto C, et al. Immunohistochemical studies of epithelial cell proliferation and p53 mutation in bovine ocular squamous cell carcinoma. Vet Pathol 2005;42:66–73.
2. Dennis MW, Lueker DC, Kainer RA. Host response to bovine ocular squamous cell carcinoma. Am J Vet Res 1985;46:1975–9.

3. Hamir AN, Parry OB. An abattoir study of bovine neoplasms with particular reference to ocular squamous cell carcinoma in Canada. Vet Rec 1980;106:551–3.
4. Heeney JL, Valli VEO. Bovine ocular squamous cell carcinoma: an epidemiological perspective. Can J Comp Med 1985;49:21–6.
5. Wilcock BP. The eye and ear. In: Jubb KVF, Kennedy PC, Palmer N, editors. Pathology of domestic animals. 4th edition. San Diego: Academic Press; 1993. p. 441–529.
6. Ivascu I. Occurrence of bovine eye neoplasms in some abattoirs and veterinary clinics in Transylvania. Wien Tierarztl Monatschr 1971;58:336–9.
7. Nair CKP, Sastry GA. A survey of animal neoplasms in Madras State. 1. Bovine. Indian Vet J 1954;30:325–31.
8. Cock EV. Some clinical observations on *Thelazia rhodessi* and squamous cell carcinoma in bovine eyes. Rhod Vet J 1972;2:62–3.
9. Epstein B. Isolation of bovine rhinotracheitis virus from ocular squamous cell carcinomas of cattle. Revista de Medicina Veterinaria 1972;53:105–10.
10. French GT. A clinical and genetic study of eye cancer in Hereford cattle. J Anim Sci 1959;9:578–81.
11. Spradbrow PB, Wilson BE, Hoffman D, et al. Immunotherapy of bovine ocular squamous cell carcinoma. Vet Rec 1977;100:376–8.
12. Stewart RJE, Hill FWG, Masztalerz A, et al. Treatment of ocular squamous cell carcinomas in cattle with interleukin-2. Vet Rec 2006;159:668–72.
13. Spadbrow PB, Hoffman D. Bovine ocular squamous cell carcinoma. Vet Bull 1980;50:449–59.
14. Russell WO, Wynne ED, Loquvam GS. Studies on bovine ocular squamous cell carcinoma (cancer eye). Cancer 1956;9:1–52.
15. Klein WR, Bier J, Van Dieten JS, et al. Radical surgery of bovine ocular squamous cell carcinoma (cancer eye) complications and results. Vet Surg 1984;13:236–42.
16. Priester WA, Mantel N. Occurrence of tumors in domestic animals. J Natl Cancer Inst 1971;47:1333–44.
17. Anderson DE, Skinner PE. Studies on bovine ocular squamous cell carcinoma ("cancer eye"). XI Effects of sunlight. J Anim Sci 1961;20:474–7.
18. Anderson DE. Cancer eye in cattle. Mod Vet Pract 1970;51:43–7.
19. Spradbrow PB, Samuel JL, Kelly WR, et al. Skin cancer and papillomaviruses in cattle. J Comp Pathol 1987;97:469–79.
20. Lloyd LC. Epithelial tumours of the skin of sheep. Br J Cancer 1961;15:780–9.
21. Russell WC, Brinks JS, Kainer RA. Incidence and heritability of ocular squamous cell tumors in Hereford cattle. J Anim Sci 1976;43:1156–62.
22. Knox JH, Koger M. A comparison of the production from range cows and yearling steers: occurrence of cancer eye in range cattle. J Anim Sci 1947;4:494.
23. Monlux AW, Anderson WA, Davis CL. The diagnosis of squamous cell carcinoma of the eye (cancer eye) in cattle. Am J Vet Res 1957;18:5–34.
24. Moulton JE. Tumors in domestic animals. Los Angeles: University of California Press; 1978. p. 443–51.
25. Woodward RR, Knapp B. The hereditary aspect of eye cancer in Hereford cattle. J Anim Sci 1950;9:578–81.
26. Blackwell RL, Anderson DE, Knox JH. Age incidence and heritability of cancer eye in Hereford cattle. J Anim Sci 1956;15:943–51.
27. Anderson DE. Effects of pigment on bovine ocular squamous cell carcinoma. Ann N Y Acad Sci 1963;100:436–46.

28. Anderson DE, Lush JL, Chambers D. Studies on bovine ocular squamous carcinoma ('cancer eye') II. Relationship between eyelid pigmentation and occurrence of cancer eye lesions. J Anim Sci 1977;16:739–46.
29. Den Otter W, Hill FWG, Klein WR, et al. Therapy of bovine ocular squamous-cell carcinoma with local doses of interleukin-2: 67 per cent complete regressions after 20 months of follow-up. Cancer Immunol Immunother 1995;41:10–4.
30. Teifke JP, Lohr CV. Immunohistochemical detection of P53 overexpression in paraffin wax-embedded squamous cell carcinomas of cattle, horses, cats and dogs. J Comp Pathol 1996;114:205–10.
31. Lee GA, Hirst LW. Ocular surface squamous neoplasia. Surv Ophthalmol 1995; 39:429–50.
32. Brash DE, Ziegler A, Jonason AS, et al. Sunlight and sunburn in human skin cancer: p53, apoptosis and tumor promotion. Symposium proceedings. J Invest Dermatol 1996;1:136–42.
33. Dmochowski L. Electron microscope studies of the replication of a virus isolated from bovine cancer eye lesions. Proc Am Assoc Cancer Res 1967;8:14.
34. Ford JN, Jennings PA, Spradbrow PB, et al. Evidence for papillomaviruses in ocular lesions in cattle. Res Vet Sci 1982;32:257–9.
35. Sykes JA, Dmochowski L, Staten W, et al. Bovine ocular squamous cell carcinoma. IV. Tissue culture studies of bovine ocular squamous cell carcinoma and its benign precursor lesions. J Natl Cancer Inst 1961;26:445–71.
36. Taylor RL, Hanks MA. Viral isolations from bovine eye tumors. Am J Vet Res 1969; 30:1885–6.
37. Anson MA, Benfield DA, McAdragh JP. Bovine herpesvirus-5 (DN-599)antigens in cells derived from bovine ocular squamous cell carcinoma. Can J Comp Med 1982;46:334–7.
38. Kuchroo VK, Spradbrow PB. Tumor-associated antigens in bovine ocular squamous cell carcinomas studies with sera from tumor-bearing animals. Vet Immunol Immunopathol 1985;9:23–36.
39. Roubicek CB, Ray DE. Genetic study of "cancer eye" in Hereford cows. Proc Am Soc Anim Sci 1974;25:49–51.
40. Mosunic CB, Moore PA, Paige K, et al. Effects of treatment with and without adjuvant radiation therapy on recurrence of ocular and adnexal squamous cell carcinoma in horses: 157 cases (1985–2002). J Am Vet Med Assoc 2004;225:1733–8.
41. Dugan SJ, Curtis R, Roberts S, et al. Epidemiological study of ocular/adnexal squamous cell carcinoma in horses. J Am Vet Med Assoc 1991;198:251–6.
42. Lall HK. Incidence of horn cancer in Meerut circle, Uttar Pradesh. Indian Vet J 1953;30:205–9.
43. Wernicke O. Hereditary eye carcinoma in cattle. Arch Oftalmol B Aires 1935;10: 773.
44. Anderson DE, Pope LS, Stephens D. Nutrition and eye cancer in cattle. J Natl Cancer Inst 1979;45:697–707.
45. Cordy DR. Nervous system and eye. Berkeley. In: Moulton JE, editor. Tumours in domestic animals. Los Angeles (CA): University of California Press; 1990. p. 654–60.
46. Farris HE, Fraunfelder FT. Cryosurgical treatment of ocular squamous cell carcinoma of Cattle. J Am Vet Med Assoc 1976;168:213–6.
47. Rutten VPMG, Klein WR, Jong DE, et al. Immunotherapy of bovine ocular squamous cell carcinoma by repeated intralesional injections of live bacillus Calmette-Guerin (BCG) or BCG cell walls. Cancer Immunol Immunother 1991;34: 186–90.

48. Gelatt KN, Brooks DE, Kallberg ME. Food and fiber-producing animal ophthalmology. In: Veterinary ophthalmology. 4th edition. Iowa: Blackwell Publishing; 2007. p. 1287–96.
49. Grier RL, Brewer WG Jr, Paul SR, et al. Treatment of bovine and equine ocular squamous cell carcinoma by radiofrequency hyperthermia. J Am Vet Med Assoc 1980;177:55–61.
50. Kainer RA, Stringer JM, Lueker DC. Hyperthermia for treatment of ocular squamous cell tumor in cattle. J Am Vet Med Assoc 1980;176:356–60.
51. Joyce JR. Cryosurgical treatment of tumor of horses and cattle. J Am Vet Med Assoc 1976;168:226–9.
52. Schoster JV. Using combined excision and cryotherapy to treat limbal squamous cell carcinoma. Vet Med 1992;87:357–65.
53. Stewart RJ, Masztalerz A, Jacobs JJ, et al. Local interleukin-2 and interleukin-12 therapy of bovine ocular squamous cell carcinomas. Vet Immunol Immunopathol 2005;106:277–84.
54. Den Otter W, De Groot JW, Bernsen MR, et al. Optimal Regimes for local IL-2 tumor therapy. Int J Cancer 1996;66:400–3.
55. Hill FWG, Klein WR, Hoyer MJ, et al. Antitumor effect of locally injected low doses of recombinant human interleukin-2 in bovine vulval papilloma and carcinoma. Vet Immunol Immunopathol 1994;41:19–29.
56. Welker B, Modransky PD, Hoffsis GF, et al. Excision of neoplasms of the bovine lower eyelid by H-blepharoplasty. Vet Surg 1991;20:133–9.
57. Bier J, Kleinschuster SJ, Corbett R. Radical surgery of bovine ocular squamous cell carcinoma: a new procedure. Vet Sci Comm 1979;3:221–30.
58. Kleinschuster SJ, Bier J, Rapp HJ, et al. Intratumoral BCG cell-wall preparation therapy and surgery in bovine ocular carcinoma. Head Neck Surg 1983;5:401–9.
59. Theilen GH, Madewell BR. Tumors of the skin. In: Theilen GH, Madewell BR, editors. Veterinary cancer medicine. Philadelphia: Lea & Febiger; 1979. p. 136–7.
60. Witrow SJ. General principles of cryosurgical technique. Vet Clin North Am Small Anim Pract 1980;10:779–86.
61. Crile G. Selective destruction of cancers after exposure to heat. Ann Surg 1962;156:404–7.
62. Muckle D, Dickson J. The selective inhibitory effect of hyperthermia on the metabolism and growth of malignant cells. Br J Cancer 1972;25:771–8.
63. Thrall DE, Gillette EL, Bauman CL. Effect of heat on the C3H mouse mammary adenocarcinoma evaluated in terms of tumor growth. Eur J Cancer 1973;9:871–5.
64. Hoffmann D, Jennings PA, Spradbrow PB. Immunotherapy of bovine ocular squamous cell carcinomas with phenol-saline extracts of allogenic carcinomas. Aust Vet J 1981;57:159–62.
65. Kainer RA. Current concepts in the treatment of bovine ocular squamous cell tumors. Vet Clin North Am Large Anim Pract 1984;6:609–22.
66. Klein WR, Ruitenberg EJ, Steerenberg PA, et al. Immunotherapy by intralesional injection of BCG walls or live BCG in bovine ocular squamous cell carcinoma: a preliminary report. J Natl Cancer Inst 1982;69:1095–101.
67. Kleinschuster SJ, Rapp HJ, Green SB, et al. Efficacy of intratumorally administered mycobacterial cell wall in the treatment of cattle with ocular carcinoma. J Natl Cancer Inst 1981;67:1165–9.
68. Kleinschuster SJ, Rapp HJ, Leukar DC, et al. Regression of bovine ocular carcinoma by treatment with a mycobacterial vaccine. J Natl Cancer Inst 1977;38:1807–14.

69. Ribi E, Ward JK, Schwartzman SM, et al. Immunotherapy of ocular squamous cell carcinoma in cattle using a mycobacterial biologic. Mod Vet Pract 1986;67: 451–3.
70. Den Otter W, Dobrowolski Z, Bugajski A, et al. Intravesical interleukin-2 in T1 papillary bladder carcinoma: regression of marker lesion in 8 of 10 patients. J Urol 1998;159:1183–6.
71. Balemans LT, Steerenberg PA, Koppenhagen FJ, et al. PEG-IL-2 therapy of advanced cancer in the guinea pig. Impact of the primary tumor and beneficial effect of cyclophosphamide. Int J Cancer 1994;58:871–6.
72. Spoormakers TJ, Klein WR, Jacobs JJ, et al. Comparison of the efficacy of local treatment of equine sarcoids with IL-2 or cisplatin/IL-2. Cancer Immunol Immunother 2003;52:179–84.
73. Bernsen MR, Van Der Velden AW, Everse LA, et al. Interleukin-2: hope in cases of cisplatin-resistant tumours. Cancer Immunol Immunother 1998;46:41–7.
74. Janeway CA, Travers P, Walport M, et al. The immune system in health and disease. London: Elsevier Science; 1999.
75. Den Otter W, Hill FWG, Klein WR, et al. Low doses of interleukin-2 can cure large bovine ocular squamous cell carcinoma. Anticancer Res 1993;13:2453–6.
76. Rutten VPMG, Klein WR, De Jong WAC, et al. Local interleukin-2 therapy in bovine ocular squamous cell carcinoma. Cancer Immunol Immunother 1989;30: 165–9.
77. Rosenberg SA, Lotze MT, Muul L, et al. A progress report on the treatment of 157 patients with advanced cancer using lymphokine activated killer cells and interleukin-2 or high dose interleukin-2 alone. N Engl J Med 1987;316:889–97.
78. Banks WC, England RB. Radioactive gold in the treatment of ocular squamous cell carcinoma of cattle. J Am Vet Med Assoc 1973;163:745–8.
79. Dugan SJ, Roberts SM, Curtis CR, et al. Prognostic factors and survival of horses with ocular/adnexal squamous cell carcinoma: 147 cases (1978–1988). J Am Vet Med Assoc 1991;198:298–303.
80. Talbot AN. Complications of beta ray treatment of pterygia. Trans Ophthalmol Soc N Z 1979;31:62–3.
81. Moore CP, Corwin LA, Collier LL. Keratopathy induced by beta radiation therapy in a horse. Equine Vet J Suppl 1983;2:112–6.
82. Merriam GR. The effects of beta radiation on the eye. Radiology 1956;66:240–4.
83. Tarr KH, Constable IJ. Late complications of pterygium treatment. Br J Ophthalmol 1980;54:496–505.
84. Tarr KH, Constable IJ. Radiation damage after pterygium treatment. Trans Ophthalmol Soc N Z 1981;33:139–42.
85. Candline FT, Levine MH. The use of beta radiation on corneal lesions in the dog. North Am Vet 1952;33:632–9.
86. Wyn-Jones G. Treatment of equine cutaneous neoplasia by radiotherapy using iridium 192 linear sources. Equine Vet J 1983;15:361–5.
87. Rehbun WC. Tumors of the eye and ocular adnexal tissues. Vet Clin North Am Equine Pract 1998;14:579–605.
88. Theon AP. Radiation therapy in the horse. Vet Clin North Am Equine Pract 1998; 14:673–89.

Ophthalmology of South American Camelids

Juliet R. Gionfriddo, DVM, MS

KEYWORDS

• Llama • Alpaca • Eye

In the past 10 years, information about South American camelid anatomy, physiology, medicine, and surgery has increased exponentially,[1] including information about the eye. In a 1997 retrospective study using the Veterinary Medical Database (VMDB) we reported that not much was known about camelid eyes but that it seemed that their eyes were not highly susceptible to disease except for trauma.[2] Although trauma-related diseases remain the most common eye problems for which camelids are presented to veterinarians, there have recently been many anecdotal reports and published case reports of camelids having ocular malignancies and potentially hereditary ocular abnormalities. The increased number of ocular diseases being reported may be because of increased recognition of camelid diseases or because of an increase in these diseases as a result of restricted gene pools as a consequence of inbreeding.

As the popularity of camelids in the world, especially in North America, is steadily increasing, owners are becoming more knowledgeable about their animals, and thus there is more need for veterinarians who understand their ocular anatomy, physiology, disease susceptibility, and recommended treatments. The purpose of this article is to provide the relevant information about the eye.

ANATOMY AND PHYSIOLOGY

The eyes of camelids are large in proportion to their head size. Their eyes are only slightly smaller than those of horses or cows even although their heads and bodies are considerably smaller. The appearance of a large eye is accentuated because they are prominently placed on the sides of the head and are framed with long eyelashes and 3 pairs of vibrissae (tactile hairs). In addition, camelid eyelids fit tightly on their globes, and cover much of the sclera so almost no white is showing. This characteristic makes the cornea seem large. The sclera and exposed conjunctiva may be

Department of Clinical Sciences, College of Veterinary Medicine and Biomedical Sciences, Veterinary Medical Center, Colorado State University, 300 West Drake Road, Fort Collins, CO 80538, USA
E-mail address: gionfri@colostate.edu

Vet Clin Food Anim 26 (2010) 531–555
doi:10.1016/j.cvfa.2010.08.004
0749-0720/10/$ – see front matter © 2010 Elsevier Inc. All rights reserved.

largely pigmented or nonpigmented, but there always seems to be a darkly pigmented, 2- to 3-mm band at the limbus. This band may protect their eyes from solar radiation damage.

The camelid eyelid is unique among domestic mammals in that there are no meibomian gland duct openings on the eyelid margins and no meibomian glands within the eyelids. Sebaceous glands on the nictitating membrane and caruncle probably fulfill the tear-layer-producing function of the meibomian glands of other species[3] (Richard Dubielzig, Diplomate American College of Veterinary Pathologists [ACVP], Madison, WI, USA, unpublished data, 2009).

The camelid has 2 nasolacrimal puncta; one is on the upper and one on the lower eyelid. These puncta are in the conjunctiva, 4 to 6 mm from the medial canthus. They are large and slitlike and are easy to cannulate. The puncta are connected to the lacrimal sac via 2 canaliculi. The nasolacrimal ducts begin in the lacrimal sac, and then run through the lacrimal and maxillary bones, across the nasal cavity, and terminate in the nasal cavity (**Figs. 1** and **2**). This nasal opening is 1.5 to 2 cm proximal to the wings of the nares and placed laterally. In the adult llama, the duct is 11 to 15 cm long and 2 to 4 mm in diameter.[4]

The corneas of llamas and alpacas are large and oval. The corneal diameters in these 2 species are similar although alpacas' heads are smaller. In one study the mean horizontal corneal diameter of llamas was 28.2 mm, whereas that of alpacas was 30.2 mm.[5] The mean vertical diameters were 24.2 mm in llamas and 22.2 mm in alpacas. The mean corneal thicknesses were also similar: measured by

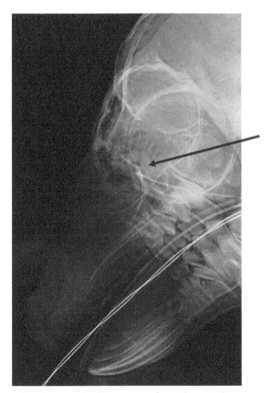

Fig. 1. Lateral view of a dacryocystorhinogram of an alpaca. The arrow is pointing to the dye in the nasolacrimal sac.

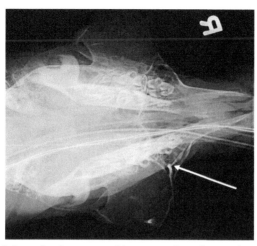

Fig. 2. Dorsoventral view of a dacryocystorhinogram of an alpaca. The arrow is pointing to the dye in the nasolacrimal sac.

ultrasonographic pachymetry, they were 608 μm in llamas and 595 μm in alpacas. Both the thicknesses and corneal diameters increased significantly with the increasing ages of the animals (juvenile vs adult animals).[5]

The corneal endothelium of camelids may be different from many other mammalian species, which may make the camelid cornea vulnerable to developing corneal edema as a result of trauma, uveitis, and surgery. Corneal edema in camelids may be profound, doubling the thickness of the cornea in some cases. At one time it was believed that camelids had fewer corneal endothelial cells (which are principally responsible for fluid removal from the cornea) than other species that are not so susceptible to corneal edema (eg, dogs and horses). However, a recent study showed that the numbers of endothelial cells in camelids (2673 cells/mm^2 in llamas and 2275 cells/mm^2 in alpacas) are only slightly lower than those of other species.[5] In that study the investigators observed frequent polymegathism (variability in cell size) and pleomorphism (variability in shape) of the endothelial cells of normal camelids, which suggested that even normal animals had corneal endothelial instability. This characteristic could make these species vulnerable to endothelial damage, with consequent corneal edema.[5]

The iris of camelids is unusual and is an adaptation for protecting the globe from excessive light exposure. On the dorsal and ventral margins of the pupil, the posterior pigment epithelium of the iris is proliferated and folded vertically. These pupillary ruffs resemble the corpora nigra of horses but are larger and consist of folded pigmented epithelial layers rather than globular masses (**Fig. 3**). In this way the ruff acts as an efficient minivisor for the eye. The iris pigmentation is usually dark, with various shades of brown scattered through an individual iris. It can also be color-dilute and can appear clear blue, gray, or have heterochromia iridis (blue and black in the same iris). A persisting rumor that blue-eyed llamas are blind has recently been refuted.[6]

The fundus of camelids may be brown, red-brown, or nonpigmented (**Figs. 4–7**). It frequently has streaks of pigment in some areas, whereas other areas in the same fundus are nonpigmented. The red coloration of the fundus that is seen in many camelids is caused by choroidal vessels that are visible through areas of nonpigmented choroid. The fundus and iris coloration are directly related to the coat and skin color of the camelid.[7] Hypopigmented animals with light coat colors generally have various

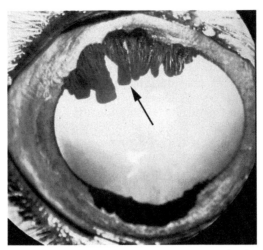

Fig. 3. The dilated pupil of an alpaca. The arrow is pointing to the dorsal papillary ruff.

combinations of gray, blue, and brown irides and reduced pigmentation of the fundus. Animals with dark coat colors generally have brown irides and pigmented fundi.[7]

The optic disk and retinal vasculature of the camelid are similar to those of the bovine and both have a holangiotic pattern (see **Figs. 4–7**). A large Bergmeister papilla (hyaloid remnant) may protrude from the disk, and 3 to 5 pairs of large, prominent, retinal vessels emerge from its periphery. One pair of vessels emerges dorsally and extends peripherally, with the artery and vein spiraling around each other. Two pairs of vessels leave the optic disk horizontally and are usually accompanied by myelin, which extends several disk diameters peripherally into the fundus.

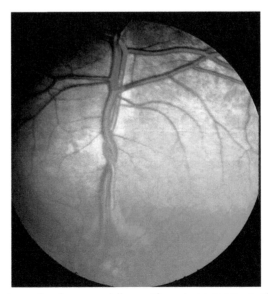

Fig. 4. Fundic photograph of a normal llama. There is no tapetum, the choroid is pigmented, and the vascular pattern is holangiotic. Note the large vessels dorsal to the optic disk and how the veins wind around each other.

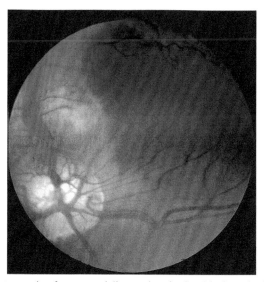

Fig. 5. Fundic photograph of a normal llama that had a black-and-white haircoat. The choroid is variably pigmented and the choroid is visible as an orange-red area dorsal to the optic disc.

The bony orbit in the skull of camelids is complete, which provides for much ocular protection. The orbit is comprised of the frontal, lacrimal, zygomatic, maxillary, palatine, temporal, and sphenoid bones. There is a large dorsal notch in the frontal bone that is palpable in living animals (**Fig. 8**). Rostral to the medial aspect of the orbit is a 2-cm-diameter opening into the nasal cavity. This opening is probably associated with a scent gland.

Vision in llamas seems to be different from that of alpacas. A report published in 2000 in which llamas and alpacas were refracted to assess their degrees of

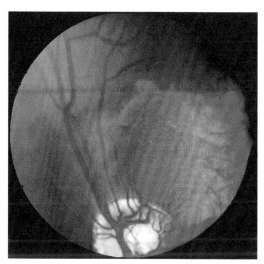

Fig. 6. Fundic photograph of a normal llama that had a white haircoat with blotches of black. The choroid is variably pigmented and is also visible as a red-orange area.

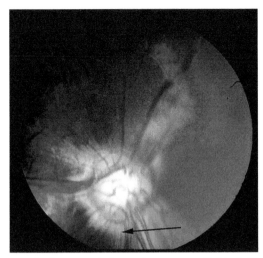

Fig. 7. Fundic photograph of a normal alpaca that was mostly black. The arrow is pointing to an area where the myelin around the optic nerve is extending around the ganglion cell axons around the optic disc.

accommodation showed that llamas are mildly myopic (nearsighted) and have some astigmatism, whereas alpacas are close to emmetropic.[8] Female llamas seem to be slightly more myopic than males. The reason for these differences is unknown but may be related to ocular size differences (eg, axial length and corneal curvature). What these values mean for the behaviors of these animals is not known. Both llama and alpacas are dichromatic in that they only see shades of blue, yellow, and gray.

EXAMINATION

A complete ocular evaluation is important in all llamas and alpacas as part of a routine physical examination and is critical when ophthalmic or systemic disease is present (**Fig. 9**). Many systemic diseases of camelids have ophthalmic manifestations, and an ocular examination can provide clues as to the nature and extent of these diseases (Richard Dubielzig, Diplomate ACVP, Madison, WI, USA, unpublished data, 2009).

Ocular examination is optimally undertaken with the llama restrained in stocks although some can be examined in a stall in a cushed position. Most camelids are

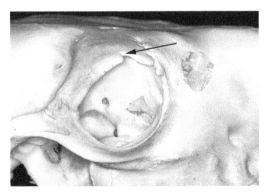

Fig. 8. The skull of a llama showing the complete bony orbit. The arrow is pointing to a palpable notch on the dorsal rim of the orbit.

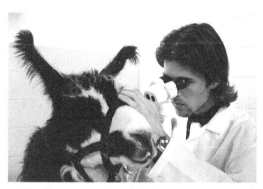

Fig. 9. Examination of the llama eye using a biomicroscope to magnify the anterior ocular structures and the eyelids. (*Courtesy of* Dr Enry Garcia da Silva, Fort Collins, CO, USA.)

amenable to examination; however, chemical sedation (butorphanol, 0.02 to 0.04 mg/kg) may be necessary to control head movement.[9,10] It is important to have diagnostic eyedrops such as tropicamide (to dilate the pupil), topical anesthetic, and fluorescein stain present when examining the eye. If the animal is in pain, topical anesthetics greatly assist the examiner to open the eye. These anesthetics may be applied to the eye via a squirt gun made from a 1- or 3-ml syringe to which a needle hub has been attached. The needle hub may be made by carefully breaking off the sharp shaft of the needle.

The examination should include complete external eye, anterior segment, and fundic examinations. The anterior portion of the eye may be examined by using magnification (such as a head loupe or slit lamp) and a bright light source. A transilluminator or halogen penlight is recommended, because regular penlights are not bright enough to elicit pupillary light reflexes (PLRs). PLRs and menace reflex responses should be elicited and Schirmer tear tests should be performed before administration of any drops. Direct and indirect PLRs of camelids are slow, and movement of the iris is minimal. The menace reflex for testing vision may be elicited by a sudden hand movement across the visual axis, and the animal should blink, retract its head, or jump back. Care must be taken not to touch or move air across the sensitive vibrasse surrounding the eye, because this elicits a false-positive response. In New World camelids the mean Schirmer tear test value is 19 mm/min in a nonanesthetized eye.[9,10] Tear production is slow in a stressed animal and obtaining an accurate measurement often requires the tear test strip to be in place for the entire minute. To test the efficiency of the lacrimal drainage system, a large amount of concentrated fluorescein dye is applied to the cornea. If the nasolacrimal system is patent, green stain may appear at the nostril within a few minutes. The same drops of stain also dye corneal ulcers.

Applanation tonometry with either a TonoPen (Mentor Ophthalmics Inc, Norwell, MA, USA) or TonoVet (Icare Finland, Helsinki, Finland) is the easiest and most accurate way of measuring intraocular pressures (IOPs) in camelids. In one study IOPs taken with a TonoPen showed that there were no differences between llamas and alpacas and that the mean IOP was 16.5 ± 3.5 mm Hg (range 14.89–18.21 mm Hg).[11] However, in a survey of camelids in Canada published in 2006 significant differences were found in IOP between the 2 species. In that study llamas had significantly lower IOPs than alpacas (mean IOP in 33 llama eyes was 16 mm Hg ± 5; mean IOP in 46 alpaca eyes was 19 mm Hg ± 4).[6] This difference between the species was believed to be because the llamas in the study were older than the alpacas and IOPs decrease as llamas and alpacas age.[11]

Mydriasis is important to conduct ophthalmoscopy effectively. To obtain mydriasis one application (about 0.2 mL) of 1% tropicamide acts within 20 to 45 minutes and lasts for about 2 hours. Indirect ophthalmoscopy using a 20-diopter lens and a trans-illuminator provides the magnified view of the fundus that is the most easy to interpret. Direct ophthalmoscopy provides for a 15-times magnification, which is good for examining details but provides only a small field of view and the observer can see only a small fundic area at one time (eg, about one-quarter of the large optic disc of camelids).

Several imaging techniques have been used to diagnose ocular and periocular diseases in camelids, including plain film radiographs, contrast radiographs, magnetic resonance imaging (MRI), computed tomography (CT), and ocular ultrasound. Dacryo-cystorhinography (see **Figs. 1** and **2**) may be used for detailed examination of the nasolacrimal drainage system. For this procedure, about 5 mL of a sodium and meglu-mine diatrizoate mixture is injected into the dorsal lacrimal punctum, and lateral and dorsoventral radiographs are then taken.[12] Alternatively, the dye can be tracked with fluoroscopy as it moves through the nasolacrimal drainage pathway. These techniques are useful for locating the site of a blockage of the nasolacrimal duct (see **Figs. 1** and **2**).[12] Ocular ultrasonography was essential for detecting the presence of a patent hyaloid artery in a llama with cataracts and is recommended before cataract surgery in camelids.[13] Ultrasound has been used to detect and characterize intraocular and ret-robulbar masses.[14,15] MRI and CT are also useful techniques for assessing retrobulbar lesions in camelids.

Medications

Most topical ocular medications that are used in other species can be used in camel-ids as well. However, care must be taken when using topical corticosteroids in these species. A recent study showed that one drop 3 times daily of topical dexamethasone-containing ophthalmic preparation for 8 days in the late stages of pregnancy could lead to abortion in llamas (Bradley Graham, DVM, Diplomate American College of Veterinary Ophthalmologists [ACVO], Denver, CO, USA, unpublished data, 2004). The delivery of topical ocular medications can be challenging. Ointments can be used by placing them directly on the cornea, or on the palpebral conjunctiva, but care must be taken to avoid touching the cornea with the tip of the ointment tube. The squirt gun method used to deliver diagnostic drops can also be used to medicate camelids. If any long-term medications are to be used the animal rapidly learns to run away or becomes fractious. This method can be wasteful of expensive drugs.

For long-term medications an ocular lavage system can be used. This system can be either through a nasolacrimal lavage tubing or through a subpalpebral lavage system (SPLS). The nasolacrimal system involves using a soft tubing (such as 22-gauge polyethelene), which is threaded into the nasal opening and up the nasolacrimal duct. The tubing stops at about the level of the nasolacrimal sac. The opposite end of the tubing is then brought out directly through the nostril, or through a needle puncture that is made in the skin of the nose, and fastened via tape tabs to the face. An injection port is then placed into the end of the tubing and injected medication can progress through the tubing, through the canaliculus, and into the eye through the punctum. Although this method is effective, it has drawbacks in that the animal must be heavily sedated to place the tubing and the tubing that exits the nose is vulnerable to being rubbed out by the animal. This medication delivery system also is not efficient because much of the injected material comes back out through the nose.

Borkowski and colleagues[16] recently reported the adaption of a commercially avail-able equine SPLS (**Fig. 10**) to deliver constant topical therapy to the eyes of 2 llamas

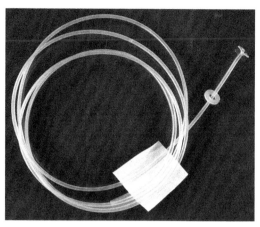

Fig. 10. SPLS that is packaged for use in horses. The round footplate in the right of the photograph is soft and is placed high in the upper palpebral fornix. The tubing is threaded through a needle puncture in the upper eyelid, continued down the neck, and an injection port is placed in the end of the tubing. This procedure allows for injection of medications. (*Courtesy of* Dr Glenn Severin, Fort Collins, CO, USA.)

with severe corneal ulcers. Initially, these systems were placed in the superior conjunctival sac in the same manner as in horses and medication was manually injected through the tubing. When the ulcers failed to heal readily it was decided that overnight delivery of medications to the eye would be beneficial. Thus, the device was modified to connect with a balloon infusion system. This system involved placing a commercial balloon infusor and flow-control tubing to the distal end of the lavage tubing. The system delivered medication at a constant rate of 1 mL/h. In each case the ulcer healed well, and the lavage system was removed within a few weeks of placement. The primary objection to using SPLSs in camelids is that camelids' tight-fitting eyelids and the lack of abundant space in the fornix could lead to rubbing of the anchoring footplate on the cornea. However, this was not a problem in the 2 llamas and the only condition associated with the system was mild swelling and irritation of one eyelid at the site of the penetration of the SPLS tubing.[16]

CAMELID OCULAR DISEASE

Reports of ocular diseases in camelids are increasing. In 1995 Gelatt and colleagues[7] described the results of ophthalmic examinations of 29 apparently healthy alpacas in South America. Although these animals had no reported clinical signs of eye problems, it was discovered that 38% of them had at least one ocular abnormality, such as conjunctivitis, corneal scars, posterior synechiae, cataracts, a subluxated lens, vitreous opacities, and/or an optic disk coloboma. Many lesions were believed to be secondary to trauma, but some may have been hereditary.[7]

In 1997 we published a retrospective study describing ocular lesions in llamas in North America. These animals had been presented to veterinary teaching hospitals in the United States and Canada over a 13-year period.[2] In 6% (194 of 3243) of the llamas seen, at least one ocular problem was diagnosed. Trauma was also considered to be the primary cause in many of these cases.

Recently a report of ophthalmic findings and hearing abilities in a group of 17 llamas and 23 alpacas living in eastern Canada was published.[6] This study was performed to examine the possible increased incidence of genetic problems in Canadian camelids as a result of the closure of the Canadian registry of llamas and alpacas to newly imported animals, which limited their gene pools. This study found that many of the animals had potentially hereditary ocular abnormalities, including persistent pupillary membranes (PPMs) (14 of 17 llamas and 5 of 23 alpacas), cataracts (9 of 17 llamas and 5 of 23 alpacas), and anterior stromal corneal dystrophy (2 of 23 alpacas). In the same study 25 llamas and 38 alpacas were tested for deafness by brainstem auditory-evoked response and the results of these tests were compared with coat and iris color. Seven of 10 pure white, blue-eyed animals were bilaterally deaf and 1 was unilaterally deaf. The investigators concluded that there was an association between skin and iris hypopigmentation and congenital sensorineural deafness in llamas and alpacas.[6]

Examination of the database at the Cooperative Ophthalmic Pathology Laboratory of Wisconsin (COPLOW), which is housed at the University of Wisconsin, showed that from 1990 to December 2009, 35 enucleated camelid eyes had been presented for histopathologic evaluation (Richard Dubielzig, Diplomate ACVP, Madison, WI, USA, unpublished data, 2009). Twenty-two of these eyes were from llamas, 12 were from alpacas, and 1 was from a guanaco. These eyes had a broad range of ophthalmic disorders. Five eyes were from crias less than 2 months of age that had various congenital disorders, whereas the rest of the disorders were either infectious, traumatic, or age-related problems. These diagnoses are discussed further in the next sections.

Congenital Diseases

Congenital nasolacrimal duct disorders seem to be common in camelids, especially alpacas. Clinical cases of these disorders usually present with a history of a wet face caused by the tears spilling out of the eye, a mucopurulent ocular discharge caused by a secondary dacryocystitis, or both. Affected animals are usually very young on presentation but occasionally the animal is older, because the problem has been ignored by the owner until periocular dermatitis and/or fly strike appears.

Congenital nasolacrimal defects that have been documented in camelids include nasolacrimal duct atresia, conjunctival punctal atresia, nasal punctual atresia, or combinations of these. In the VMDB database study, conjunctival nasolacrimal defects were recorded in 5 llama crias[2]; in addition, 4 llamas examined by Glenn Severin had congenital conjunctival punctal atresia (Glenn Severin, DVM, Diplomate ACVO, Fort Collins, CO, USA, personal communication, 1993). The abnormal puncta were surgically opened and catheterized using a procedure similar to that in horses.[17] Sapienza and colleagues[4] published a case of severe epiphora caused by bilateral atresia of the nasolacrimal ducts in a llama cria. In that animal the palpebral puncta were patent on both sides and the obstructions were at the nasal puncta. Surgical opening of the ducts was successful.[4]

Since the VMDB study was published, 5 cases of bilateral nasolacrimal duct obstruction have been seen in alpaca crias presented to Colorado State University (Juliet R. Gionfriddo, DVM, Diplomate ACVO, Fort Collins, CO, USA, unpublished data, 2010). Three of these were from the same alpaca farm and were distantly related. In 4 of the 5 crias the obstruction was caused by failure of the formation of the nasal punctum bilaterally. Treatment of these crias involved placing the animals under general anesthesia and catheterizing the nasolacrimal ducts through the conjunctival puncta with polyethylene tubing. On each side the tubing was threaded down the nasolacrimal duct until it stopped at the point where the duct blind-ended. In 3 of the alpaca crias the tip of the tubing could be palpated through the nasal mucosa on both sides at the point where the puncta should have been. An incision through the mucosa over the tubing was made and the tubing was passed into the nasal cavity, at which point it was anchored to the surrounding nasal mucosa with a Chinese finger knot. It was then threaded through a large needle, which was used to pierce the skin of the nares, and was attached to the skin with tape tabs. The tubing was left in place for 6 weeks so that the punctum would not close. This procedure corrected the problem in each case.

The fourth cria proved to be more difficult to treat in that the tubing could not be palpated through the nasal mucosa. A dacryocystorhinogram (see the section on ancillary diagnostic techniques) was performed and showed that the obstructions on both sides were caused by failure of formation of the distal one-third of the nasolacrimal ducts.[12] Thus, the tubing had stopped at the level of the maxillary bones. A bilateral conjunctivosinusostomy (creating a new opening from the conjunctiva into the sinus) was performed to allow for lacrimal drainage; this technique is complicated and is described in the cited paper by Mangan and colleagues[12] and discussed later in the section on dacryocystitis.

To the author's knowledge, the only reported congenital defects of the anterior segment are PPMs. Webb and colleagues[6] reported a high incidence of this defect in the 40 llamas that they examined but did not give the exact number. These PPMs were classified as iris-to-iris and were causing no visual deficits or other problems. Because these defects are hereditary in dogs, the investigators suggest that they may be hereditary in camelids as well.

Numerous camelids with congenital defects of the posterior segment have been seen[2,7,18] (Richard Dubielzig, Diplomate ACVP, Madison, WI, USA, unpublished data, 2009). These defects may be confined to a single structure such as the retina, choroid, or optic nerve or, more often, may involve multiple structures and even the entire globe. The COPLOW database reported the results of histopathologic examination of the eyes of 7 camelid crias less than 8 weeks of age (Richard Dubielzig, Diplomate ACVP, Madison, WI, USA, unpublished data, 2009). All of these had multiple ocular defects and 6 of the 7 had peripapillary colobomas. This finding suggested that there had been a failure of the closure of the fetal fissure of the eye. Two of the 7 eyes were micoophthalmic; one also had a lens rupture and the other had a coloboma and retinal dysplasia (Richard Dubielzig, Diplomate ACVP, Madison, WI, USA, unpublished data, 2009). Schuh and colleagues[18] described an adult llama with a large coloboma near the optic disk in one eye. This report, along with anecdotal reports of finding colobomas in allegedly normal adult camelids, suggests that they may be common defects in camelid eyes but may go undiagnosed because there are no other obvious visual defects. Although there are no studies documenting the potential heritability of colobomas in camelids, they are hereditary in some breeds of cattle[17] and dogs,[19] and therefore animals with this defect should either not be bred from or should be outcrossed.

Other congenital posterior segment findings in the cria eyes in the COPLOW database were a retinal detachment, in an eye that also had vitreous fibrosis and ossification, optic nerve hypoplasia, tunica vasculosa lentis, and retinal aplasia (Richard Dubielzig, Diplomate ACVP, Madison WI, USA, unpublished data, 2009). These congenital defects of camelid eyes seem to be uncommon and whether or not they are genetic in origin is unknown. None is treatable and often blindness or visual defects may be present as a result of the defect.

Acquired Diseases

Cornea

Corneal disease is probably the most frequently seen ocular abnormality in camelids. This finding is not surprising considering the prominence and potential vulnerability of this structure. Corneal trauma may be caused by fighting, penetration of the cornea with plant material, or from recumbency as a result of prolonged anesthesia, tick paralysis, meningeal worms, or lack of passive transfer in crias.[2] In studies of apparently healthy camelids having no history of squinting, many corneal scars suggestive of prior trauma were seen.[6,7] In symptomatic llamas that were presented to veterinary teaching hospitals, 41% had active corneal disease, of which more than half were ulcers (**Figs. 11** and **12**).[2] Most of these ulcers were of unknown cause but were probably traumatic in origin. Other trauma-associated corneal diseases reported in that study included lacerations, foreign bodies, and stromal abscesses.[2,9] The COPLOW database contained reports of 2 alpaca eyes that had been enucleated for corneal perforations caused by trauma; both had secondary infection (Richard Dubielzig, Diplomate ACVP, Madison, WI, USA, unpublished data, 2009). One of these eyes also had an explosive choroidal hemorrhage secondary to the perforation. One llama eye reported in the database had an extensive corneal abscess.

Abscesses seem to be a common sequela of camelid eyes to penetrating corneal trauma (Juliet R. Gionfriddo, DVM, Diplomate ACVO, Fort Collins, CO, USA, unpublished data, 2010; Richard Dubielzig, Diplomate ACVP, Madison, WI, USA, unpublished data, 2009). These abscesses appear as yellowish-white collections of purulent material at various depths in the corneal stroma; they are often deep (see **Fig. 11**). These abscesses generally are infected but unlike in horses, if they are treated aggressively they often resolve quickly. Some of these abscesses may be fungal in origin, and mycotic keratitis has been seen in several camelids (Juliet R. Gionfriddo, DVM, Diplomate ACVO, Fort Collins, CO, USA, unpublished data, 2010). Mycotic keratitis may not clear up easily because fungi tend to grow deeply into the cornea and can penetrate the globe to cause fungal enophthalmitis.

Aggressive and prompt treatment of corneal ulcers, lacerations, and abscesses in camelids is important to provide the best chance of a good outcome[9] (Juliet R. Gionfriddo, DVM, Diplomate ACVO, Fort Collins, CO, USA, unpublished data, 2009). Topical ophthalmic antibiotics should be used in all cases in which the corneal epithelium has been compromised. Bacterial cultures of normal camelid eyes (llamas, guanacos, and alpacas) grew mixed bacterial populations but many of the bacteria were identified as opportunistic pathogens. Thus topical broad-spectrum antibiotics such as a triple antibiotic ointment or ofloxacin should be used initially, and then changes in the antibiotic type can be made later if needed (Juliet R. Gionfriddo,

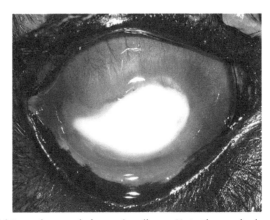

Fig. 11. Large, midstromal corneal abscess in a llama. Note the marked vascular response of the cornea to the lesion.

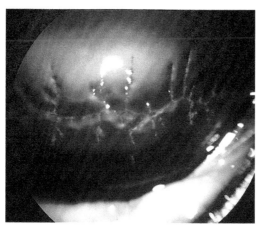

Fig. 12. Superficial dendritic ulcer in a llama cornea. This ulcer is similar to dendritic ulcers caused by herpesvirus in cats. (*Courtesy of* Dr Michael Blair, Richmond, VA, USA.)

DVM, Diplomate ACVO, Fort Collins, CO, USA, unpublished data, 2009). If the ulcer seems to be infected (eg, if it is becoming deeper or melting), initial cytology of the ulcer along with aerobic culture and sensitivities and fungal cultures should be performed and the appropriate antibiotic or antifungal drug may be chosen. All topical antibiotics that can be used in horses can be used in camelids as well. Ofloxacin seems to be a good antibiotic choice for treatment of infected ulcers in camelids (Juliet R. Gionfriddo, DVM, Diplomate ACVO, Fort Collins, CO, USA, unpublished data, 2009).

Chronic superficial corneal defects (also called indolent or undermined ulcers) have been seen in camelids. The cause for these defects is unknown but could be the same as for dogs. Successful treatment of these defects has included debridement and removal of the superficial stroma using a diamond burr technique that has proved successful in dogs (**Fig. 13**)[20] (Juliet R. Gionfriddo, DVM, Diplomate ACVO, Fort Collins, CO, USA, unpublished data, 2009).

Recent anecdotal reports have implicated a herpesvirus as the cause of superficial, dendritic ulcers in camelids (Ursula Dietrich, Diplomate ACVO, Athens, GA, USA, personal communication, 2009; Michael J. Blair, DVM, MS, Diplomate ACVO, Richmond, VA, USA, personal communication, 2009; Juliet R. Gionfriddo, DVM, Diplomate ACVO, Fort Collins, CO, USA, unpublished data, 2009). These ulcers seem to be similar to those in cats but as of yet the organism has not been positively detected. Studies are under way to attempt this (Juliet R. Gionfriddo, DVM, Diplomate ACVO, Fort Collins, CO, USA, unpublished data, 2009). The fact that these corneal ulcers generally heal well if the animal is placed on eyedrops containing cidofovir suggests that they may be at least viral in origin.

There have been several anecdotal reports and one published case report of camelids with corneal degeneration. An alpaca with a history of cloudy corneas and decreased vision was presented to the Veterinary Teaching Hospital of Zurich.[21] The corneas had fluorescein-positive erosions that were surrounded by areas of neovascularization and dense-white crystalline deposits. A diagnosis of bilateral lipid keratopathy was made based on the clinical signs and results of histopathologic examination of the portions of the corneas that were removed with a superficial keratectomy. The alpaca had high serum cholesterol concentrations, which probably led to lipid deposition in the corneas of this animal.[21]

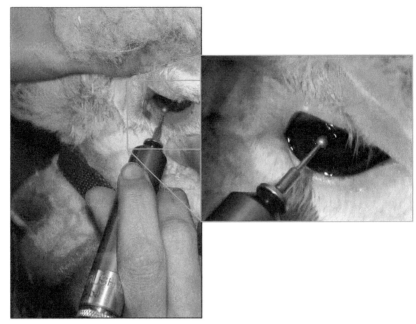

Fig. 13. The diamond burr procedure being used to debride and polish a chronic superficial ulcerative lesion on the cornea of an alpaca. (*Courtesy of* Dr Enry Garcia da Silva, Fort Collins, CO, USA.)

Treatment of corneal lacerations, deep ulcers, or perforations depends on the initial depth of the lesion (eg, full thickness versus superficial), the skills of the clinician, the desires of the owner, the duration of the problem, and whether or not the lesion is infected. Greater than half-depth lacerations that have little to no corneal tissue missing may be sutured directly with small-gauge (6-0 to 8-0), absorbable, suture material such as Prolene (Ethicon Inc, Auneau, France). Deep ulcers and ulcers with perforations may be successfully repaired using a conjunctival pedicle graft. Rodriguez-Alvaro and colleagues[22] reported on an adult alpaca in the Zoo-Aquarium in Madrid that had a corneal perforation with a prolapsed iris. This condition was repaired with a bulbar conjunctival pedical graft that, after amputation of the protruding iris, was sutured to the cornea with 6-0 Vicryl in a simple interrupted pattern. During the surgery the alpaca was paralyzed with atricurium and the anterior chamber was maintained with viscoelastic. The animal recovered well and had vision in the eye.[22] All that remained long-term was a corneal scar and dyscoria. Grafting techniques are technically difficult and require the use of an operating microscope. Therefore animals needing grafts should be referred to a veterinary ophthalmologist for optimal care.

Other corneal diseases reported in camelids include dystrophies, degenerations, dermoids, and edema[2,23] (Glenn A. Severin, DVM, Diplomate ACVO, Fort Collins, CO, USA, personal communication, 1993). Bilateral, spontaneous, corneal edema was reported in a guanaco and her offspring.[23] The cause was not found. Although the number of corneal endothelial cells of llamas and alpacas is comparable with that of other species,[5] the cells may be sensitive to insults and, if damaged, may become ineffective in removing excess water from the corneal stroma. Although endothelial protective measures during intraocular surgeries have been instituted,[24] corneal edema can still develop after intraocular surgery and corneal trauma in camelids.

Conjunctiva

Conjunctivitis is common in camelids and the clinical signs include mild squinting, conjunctival hyperemia, and epiphora (**Fig. 14**). Elevation of the eyelids reveals conjunctival hyperemia and possibly chemosis. In these cases the conjunctival sac (including the section on the third eyelid) should be carefully inspected for foreign material or lymphoid follicle development. Most conjunctivitis cases are caused by irritation (eg, wind, dust, foreign bodies) and are self limiting if the offending irritant is removed.

In the VMDB study, diseases of the conjunctiva were reported in 19 llamas (10% of the llamas with ocular disease).[2] Most of these cases were conjunctivitis due to unknown cause, and were probably caused by irritation but there were several cases of conjunctival infection.[2] Clinical signs of bacterial conjunctivitis are more severe than those caused by irritation and often include marked hyperemia, mucopurulent ocular discharge, and blepharospasm (see **Fig. 14**). A variety of bacterial species have been isolated from llamas with severe conjunctivitis and these were suspected to be the primary cause of the disease (although they could have been secondary invaders) (Juliet R. Gionfriddo, DVM, Diplomate ACVO, Fort Collins, CO, USA, unpublished data, 1990). Brightman and colleagues[25] reported a case of keratoconjunctivitis in a llama from which *Staphylococcus aureus* was isolated. Microbiologic culture (both bacterial and fungal) and sensitivity testing are recommended in most cases of conjunctivitis and keratoconjunctivitis. Most bacterial infections respond well to appropriate topical antibacterial therapy.

Conjunctivitis in camelids may also be caused by chlamydiae (Glenn A. Severin, DVM, Diplomate ACVO, Fort Collins, CO, USA, personal communication, 1993) and parasites. *Thelazia californiensis*, a nematode, has been found in the conjunctival sac of many species, including llamas.[26] Symptoms of *Thalezia* conjunctivitis range from those of mild epiphora and hyperemia to severe epiphora and blepharospasm (if ulcerative keratitis also occurs).[26] The initial signs of infection are usually those of nonspecific conjunctivitis. This larval nematode is transmitted between animals by face flies, and may be seen moving across the surface of the eye or hiding beneath the third eyelid. Treatment consists of mechanical removal following topical anesthesia, or topical diethylcarbamazine or ivermectin instilled into the conjunctival sac to kill the parasite.[26]

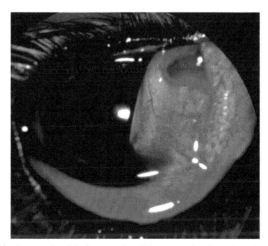

Fig. 14. The eye of a 3-month-old alpaca cria with severe bacterial conjunctivitis. A *Streptococcus* organism was cultured from the eye.

Many types of flies feed on llama lacrimal secretions and can cause conjunctival irritation. Consequently, fly control is important for minimizing this form of conjunctivitis.

Noninfectious conjunctival abnormalities include trauma, foreign bodies, dermoids, and congenital cysts.[2,18,26] Large conjunctival wounds should be sutured with small-gauge (eg, 5-0), absorbable suture material. Small wounds usually heal with medical therapy alone. Congenital cysts have been reported infrequently in neonatal crias.[18] Schuh and colleagues[18] reported a cystlike structure on the bulbar conjunctiva of a cria. Aspiration of this structure yielded a clear fluid. Because the same eye had other defects, the cyst was believed to be part of a general ocular maldevelopment. A conjunctival cyst, without other ocular lesions, was reported by Johnson (LaRue Johnson, DVM PhD, Fort Collins, CO, USA, personal communication, 1999). Drainage of the cyst failed to permanently resolve the problem but surgical excision proved curative.

Eyelid, nictitating membrane, and nasolacrimal system

The incidence of eyelid lesions in llamas and alpacas seems to be low. In the VMDB study only 13 llamas were reported to have eyelid diseases.[2] Blepharitis was the most common eyelid problem, and these cases were often seen in conjunction with generalized dermatitis. Blepharitis caused by bacterial infection has been seen and often occurs along with bacterial conjunctivitis.[2] Few reports exist of eyelid lacerations in camelids and in the VMDB study; they were seen in only 2 llamas.[2] However, full-thickness eyelid lacerations can be serious because of the potential for secondary corneal damage from exposure of the globe and therefore they should be sutured. Because the camelid eyelids fit so closely on the cornea, great care must be taken to avoid exposure of the suture or knots to the corneal surface. All full-thickness lacerations should be sutured in a 2-layer closure; the first layer should be in the muscle and the second in the skin.

Until recently no cases of periocular neoplasms had been reported. However, in an article on the prevalence of neoplasms in llamas and alpacas in Oregon from 2001 to 2006, Valentine and Martin[27] documented squamous cell carcinomas on the nictitating membranes of one llama and one alpaca. An ossifying fibroma originating in the area of the second premolar of a 4.5-year-old llama manifested as a firm mass near the medial canthus of the left eye was also reported.[28] Nasal endoscopy revealed a mucosa-covered mass that was originating by the tooth and extending to the soft palate. Although this mass was close to the nasolacrimal system, no epiphora was noted.[28]

Nasolacrimal disorders in camelids are mostly congenital, as discussed earlier. Dacryocystitis and inflammation of the nasolacrimal system are common, perhaps because the large conjunctival punctum is vulnerable to invasion by foreign bodies such as grass awns. Animals with this disorder are usually adults and have a history of chronic mucopurulent ocular discharge, which can be profuse. There can also be a history of squinting and conjunctival redness. Treatment of dacryocystitis is aimed at clearing the nasolacrimal system of foreign material and clearing up the secondary bacterial infection that accompanies it. Topical antibiotics can be tried initially but frequently do not clear up the problem. Flushing of the nasolacrimal duct through the upper or lower punctum often removes foreign material, pus, and infectious agents (**Fig. 15**). This procedure can often be performed with the animal awake after instillation of topical anesthetic drops. If the system does not flush easily and more aggressive flushing is necessary, general anesthetic may be needed.

Lens

Cataracts are the most common abnormalities of the camelid lens. They were reported in 20 animals (10%) in the VMDB[2,7] (Glenn A. Severin, DVM, Diplomate

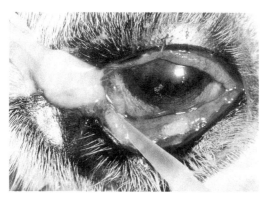

Fig. 15. Flushing the nasolacrimal sac of a llama with dacryocystitis. A soft catheter was placed in the lower punctum and the system was flushed with sterile saline. In this case a large amount of purulent material was removed from the nasolacrimal sac. Occasional plant material is flushed out of the sac as well.

ACVO, Fort Collins, CO, USA, personal communication, 1993). Mature, hypermature, and immature cataracts have been reported.[6,7,9,10,23,24,29–32] In a South American herd of 29 alpacas, Gelatt and colleagues[7] saw one animal with apparently normal vision but with nuclear cataracts. In a survey of camelids in Canada, Webb and colleagues[6] found incipient anterior cortical cataracts in 2 llamas and 3 alpacas, incipient posterior cortical cataracts in 5 llamas and 1 alpaca, and immature posterior capsular and cortical cataracts in 3 llamas. Whether these small, immature cataracts in camelids progress to maturity or whether they are inherited is unknown.[23,26,31,33] In one report of an adult alpaca with type 1 diabetes mellitus, the investigators reported that the animal had bilateral posterior lens capsule opacities that covered more than 50% of the lenses.[32] It is not known whether or not these opacities were caused by the systemic disease; however, they were dissimilar to diabetic cataracts in dogs, which develop rapidly and progress to maturity.[32]

Mature cataracts in camelids can severely impair vision, but surgical removal has proved successful in restoring vision in these species.[13,24,30] In the past, cataract removal was unsuccessful because of its severe, vision-threatening complications. In one report published in 1993 of cataract surgery in a llama, lens extraction was followed by severe corneal edema, ulcerative keratitis, and phthisis bulbi.[31] The use of advanced phacoemulsification techniques, endothelial protective viscoelastics during surgery, special endothelial protective irrigating solutions, and the extensive use of antiinflammatory drugs have improved the success rate of cataract removal in camelids.[13,24] To the author's knowledge no intraocular lens placement has been attempted in camelids.

In one report of cataract surgery in a 9-month-old female llama, a persistent hyperplastic primary vitreous, persistent tunica vasculosa lentis and persistent hyaloid artery (filled with blood) were present in the right eye. These conditions were not discovered until the lens had been removed during surgery.[13] Color Doppler ultrasound performed before surgery in the left eye of the llama showed that there was a patent tunica vasculosa lentis in that eye as well. Despite these complications, vision was restored in both eyes of the llama. Powell and colleagues[24] reported on cataract surgery in a 14-year-old llama. The cataracts were age-related and not associated with any other ocular defects. The surgery was performed with routine phacoemulsification techniques. Although the surgery went smoothly, the llama developed severely increased IOPs postoperatively. After the posterior capsule was perforated surgically, the IOPs returned to normal. The increased pressures were attributed to a possible pupillary and drainage angle blockage caused by the vitreous imbibing water and moving forward (aqueous misdirection).[24] Cataract surgery in these animals is difficult but if performed by an experienced veterinary ophthalmic surgeon the success rate is high.

Although infrequently seen, other lens diseases in llamas include luxated lenses, traumatic lens ruptures, and lens colobomas. A lens coloboma was seen temporally in the left lens of a female guanaco and was associated with nuclear and perinuclear cataracts and corneal edema.[23] A hereditary cause for the defects was suspected. In an eye of a 1-day-old cria that was recorded in the COPLOW database a lens rupture was noted. This rupture was seen in conjunction with other abnormalities such as microphthalmia and an ocular coloboma (Richard Dubielzig, Diplomate ACVP, Madison, WI, USA, unpublished data, 2009). Lens ruptures can also occur secondarily to severe ocular trauma.

Uvea

As in other species, uveitis seems to be a commonly seen sequela of systemic disease as well as of direct ocular trauma in camelids (**Figs. 16** and **17**). In the VMDB study 18% of the llamas with eye disease had uveitis.[2] Anterior uveitis has been seen in septicemic neonates and crias with juvenile llama immunodeficiency syndrome.[2] Uveitis may also be secondary to deep ulcerative keratitis, lens-induced uveitis, trauma, and infectious disease such as equine herpesvirus type 1 (EHV-1)[33-35] (Richard Dubielzig, Diplomate ACVP, Madison, WI, USA, unpublished data, 2009). EHV-1 can cause anterior uveitis, severe chorioretinitis, and neurologic disease in camelids.[33] Camelids acquire EHV-1 by contact with members of the family Equidae. A report published in 1988 described a mixed herd of camelids in which many members became blind after exposure to infected zebras.[33] Neurologic signs including head tilt, nystagmus, and paralysis developed in 4 alpacas. Ophthalmoscopy showed vitritis, retinitis, and optic neuritis. Two alpacas also had hypopyon and iritis. All attempted treatments failed to restore vision to any animal.[33] Histologic identification of eosinophilic inclusions in the brain and measurement of high EHV-1 antibody titers in the serum confirmed EHV-1 as the cause.[33] In 1989 a similar outbreak occurred in a herd of llamas in Illinois (Deborah S. Friedman, DVM, Diplomate ACVO, Fremont,

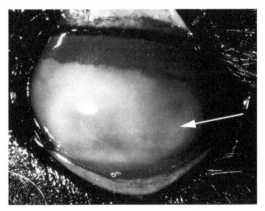

Fig. 16. A llama with severe, suppurative anterior uveitis. There is a large area of hypopion (*yellow arrow*) and a marked corneal neovascularization. The vessels are in a brush border and are small and straight, characteristic of deep vascular invasion.

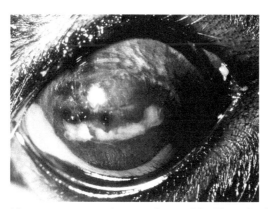

Fig. 17. A llama with severe, suppurative anterior uveitis. There is also hypopion and marked posterior synechiae. Both of the animals in **Figs. 16** and **17** had septicemia and pneumonia.

CA, USA, unpublished data, 1989). Twenty-eight llamas were exposed to zebras with rhinitis. Ten to 17 days after exposure, neurologic signs (including blindness, deafness, head tilt, and circling) developed in most of the llamas. Ophthalmic examination showed severe anterior uveitis and chorioretinitis. EHV-1 was confirmed as the cause of this outbreak (Deborah S. Friedman, DVM, Diplomate ACVO, Fremont, CA, USA, unpublished data, 1989).

House and colleagues[35] in 1991 infected 3 llamas with EHV-1. Two of the llamas exhibited severe neurologic signs, including blindness, staggering, head tremors, and depression. Histopathologic assessment showed severe neuronal changes in the brain and optic nerve. Isolation of EHV-1 was successful in only one (the most clinically ill) of the 3 infected animals, which suggests that it may be difficult to isolate the virus from infected animals.[35]

Paulsen and colleagues[34] described a llama with chorioretinitis, optic neuritis, and encephalitis. Serologic tests failed to implicate EHV-1, and no intranuclear inclusion bodies were seen histopathologically. The similarity of the clinical signs of this animal to those of the alpacas described by Rebhun and colleagues suggests that it may have been a case of chronic EHV-1, in which the virus was not identified. To the author's knowledge no outbreaks of this disease have been reported in camelids since the 1990s.

Clinical signs of uveitis can range from mild squinting, epiphora, and aqueous flare to severe pain signs, red eye, synechiae, and corneal edema. In 2001 Grahn and colleagues[36] published a case report of a 9-year-old female llama with a history of red eye of several months' duration. The llama developed photophobia and ocular discharge just before presentation. Ophthalmic examination showed bilateral focal corneal degeneration, multiple areas of anterior and posterior synechiae (with iris bombe in the right eye), and aqueous and vitreous flare. Routine blood work on the llama included a complete blood count, serum biochemical profile, and urinalysis. In addition, serum titers for Leptospirosis, Toxoplasma, Brucella abortus, and EHV were recommended but were not elected by the owners. Because the basic blood work was within normal range a diagnosis of bilateral idiopathic uveitis was made and intense antiinflammatory therapy was instituted. This therapy included oral flunixin meglumine (1 mg/kg every 24 hours for 7 days) and topical atropine, flurbiprofen, and prednisolone acetate. The llama was rechecked at 4 days and 1 month, and by the 1-month recheck the right eye was buphthalmic and had lost vision. A poor prognosis for vision was given because of the glaucoma.[36]

Camelids with uveitis that is not attributable to an obvious cause should be examined carefully for signs of systemic disease. A history should be taken, and physical and ocular examination should be performed. Routine blood work is indicated in these cases as well as serology that is appropriate for the area and physical examination findings. The diseases that are known to cause uveitis in camelids include all the ones recommended by Grahn and colleagues,[36] with the addition of regional systemic fungal organisms (eg, blastomycosis, coccidiodomycosis) and systemic aspergillosis (rare).[37]

If no cause for the uveitis can be found then one must consider a diagnosis of idiopathic uveitis, and the animal should be given antiinflammatory therapy. This therapy generally includes systemic nonsteroidal antiinflammatory drugs (NSAIDs), and topical steroids (only if no corneal ulcer is present) and/or NSAIDs. Topical atropine is also indicated to prevent synechiae and help alleviate pain.

Posterior segment: retina, optic nerve

Diseases of the posterior segment are common in camelids. Congenital abnormalities, inflammatory diseases, toxic retinopathy, and retinal and optic nerve degenerations have been noted. In the VMDB, 11 animals (6%) were reported to have retinal lesions, including retinitis, retinal detachment, retinal dystrophy, and retinal degeneration.[2] Optic nerve disease was reported in 2 llamas: 1 had optic nerve hypoplasia and the other had a coloboma. Seven cria eyes with multiple ocular defects were recorded in the COPLOW database and all of these had posterior segment abnormalities (Richard Dubielzig, Diplomate ACVP, Madison, WI, USA, unpublished data, 2009). These defects were all considered to be congenital (see section on congenital defects).

Several infectious systemic diseases have been reported to cause posterior segment inflammatory disease in camelids. The most notorious is EHV-1, as discussed earlier. Other diseases reported to lead to posterior segment inflammation in llamas include aspergillosis, toxoplasmosis, and septicemia[37,38] (David Tinsley, DVM, Diplomate ACVO, Gloucester, ON, Canada, unpublished data, 1996). Aspergillosis was implicated as a cause of neurologic disease and chorioretinitis in a wild-caught, zoo-housed alpaca.[37] During a postmortem examination, *Aspergillus* was identified in the lung and eye. The fungus was believed to have spread from the lungs to the eye hematogenously.

Toxoplasmosis, a known cause of chorioretinitis in dogs and cats, may also cause blindness in camelids (LaRue Johnson, DVM, PhD, Fort Collins, CO, USA, unpublished data, 1993; David Tinsley, DVM, Diplomate ACVO, Gloucester, ON, Canada, unpublished data, 1996). During an investigation of causes of late-term abortions in llamas, a serologic survey showed a high antibody titer for *Toxoplasma gondii* in a blind llama who did not abort (LaRue Johnson, DVM, PhD, Fort Collins, CO, USA, unpublished data, 1993). The llama had lesions of chronic panophthalmitis. Tinsley described a 15-year-old llama with signs of bilateral chorioretinitis (David Tinsley, DVM, Diplomate ACVO, Gloucester, ON, Canada, unpublished data, 1996). Vitreous humor was collected from one eye at hospital admission and 1 month later. Vitreous toxoplasmosis antibody titers showed a marked increase, although serum antibody titers were negative. These results suggested that an ocular *Toxoplasma gondii* infection may have caused the uveitis (David Tinsley, DVM, Diplomate ACVO, Gloucester, ON, Canada, unpublished data, 1996).

In a report published in 1992 about 6 camelid crias (5 llamas and 1 alpaca) that had gram-negative septicemias, only 2 crias survived.[38] After initiation of treatments for the infections one cria developed secondary, bilateral retinal detachments and chorioretinitis. Other clinical signs of the infection were depression, convulsions, diarrhea, and respiratory distress. The bacteremias were attributed to perinatal factors and poor transfer of maternal antibodies.[38]

Noninflammatory retinal diseases have been reported in camelids but these cases were congenital developmental defects, or secondary to toxicities, glaucoma, or age. To the author's knowledge, no hereditary retinal atrophic diseases such as progressive retinal atrophy have been reported in camelid species. In the COPLOW database retina aplasia or dystrophy was reported in 4 of the 7 cria eyes that had congenital defects (Richard Dubielzig, Diplomate ACVP, Madison, WI, USA, unpublished data, 2009). In adult camelid eyes in this database, retinal atrophy was reported in one 10-year-old alpaca whose eye had been enucleated as a result of chronic glaucoma. Retinal detachments were reported in 2 glaucomatous eyes in older llamas (Richard Dubielzig, Diplomate ACVP, Madison, WI, USA, unpublished data, 2009).

Harrison and colleagues reported on a possible toxic retinopathy in a zoo-housed male guanaco (a wild New World camelid that is related to llamas and alpacas).[39] The animal had an abdominal laceration, which was surgically repaired. It was treated with penicillin G procaine and benzathine and enrofloxacin (2.4 mg/kg by mouth every 24 hours for 10 days), which were begun immediately postoperatively. Later trimethoprim-sulfadiazine was added to the treatment regimen. Twenty-six days after surgery the guanaco was blind and had optic nerve pallor. The animal was killed and histopathology of its eyes showed that it had central retinal atrophy. In addition, the brain had scattered areas of neuronal necrosis, microgliosis, and cerebral edema. The investigators concluded that this was a case of enrofloxacin toxicity because of its similarity to the toxicity found in cats. However, this diagnosis could not be proven.[39]

Glaucoma

Glaucoma is not commonly seen in camelids but when it does occur it is secondary to intraocular inflammation or is congenital. No reports confirming primary, potentially hereditary, glaucoma in llamas or alpacas were found; however, there is one report of a guanaco with goniodysgenesis.[23] Barrie and colleagues used gonioscopy to examine the drainage angle of a guanaco with corneal edema but normal IOPs.[23] They found the drainage angles to be closed and spanned by uveal tissue.

Only 2 cases of glaucoma were reported in the VMDB study.[2] Later, 3 cases were found in the COPLOW database; one was secondary to lens rupture, one was caused by suppurative endophthalmisis, and one was chronic, caused by unknown inflammation. Cullen and Grahn[40] published a case report about a 6-month-old female llama that was diagnosed with congenital glaucoma. The llama had had prominent eyes, epiphora, corneal cloudiness, and angular limb deformities since birth but was not blind. Ocular examination revealed numerous anomalies including buphthalmos, corneal edema and striae, prolapsed vitreous and PPMs. The llama was killed and histopathologic examination of the globes showed iris hypoplasia and poorly developed iridocorneal angles. This condition was not believed to be hereditary because the dam and sire had been bred several times before the birth of this cria and had produced only normal animals.[40]

Despite these case reports the incidence of goniodysgenesis and subsequent glaucoma in camelids is apparently low. However, routine tonometry and gonioscopy on diseased and healthy eyes may show a higher incidence of glaucoma or goniodysgenesis than has been reported.

Visual deficits of unknown origin have been reported. Eleven blind neonatal crias with apparently normal fundi were seen at Colorado State University Veterinary Teaching Hospital over a 20-year period (Glenn A. Severin, DVM, Diplomate ACVO, Fort Collins, CO, USA, personal communication, 1993). Vision gradually returned to all crias; no cause was found. Congenital nystagmus and amblyopia have also been diagnosed in crias. There are also anecdotal reports of blindness with no apparent ocular defects or diseases in adult llamas (LaRue Johnson, DVM, PhD, Fort Collins, CO, USA, personal communication, 1999). These cases may be an undiagnosed optic nerve or brain disorder.

An electroretinogram (ERG) may be performed in blind camelids to distinguish between a retinal disorder and an optic nerve or cerebral cortical lesions. The ERG amplitude of a normal camelid is higher than that of most normal dogs and cats (Juliet R. Gionfriddo, DVM, Diplomate ACVO, Fort Collins, CO, USA, unpublished data, 2010). Visual evoked potentials can also be generated in camelids to test the visual pathways and explore the cause of the blindness.

Neoplasia

Ocular and periocular neoplasia seem to be more common in domestic camelids than previously believed. In the VMDB study published in 1997 only 2 cases of neoplasia were reported in llamas.[2] One was an intraocular medulloepithelioma and the other was an unspecified corneal tumor. Recently 5 case reports of intraocular tumors in llamas have appeared in the literature. Three of these were primitive round cell tumors derived from the inner layer of the optic cup before differentiation and were considered to be congenital tumors. This finding suggests that these types of tumors are more common than in other domestic animal species.[41] In 2000, Hendricks and colleagues[41] reported a malignant, intraocular, teratoid, medulloepithelioma in the eye of a 1-year-old llama. Presenting signs in this patient were those of anterior uveitis, blindness, and retinal detachment. Because these signs were suggestive of an infectious uveitis, blood work and serology for toxoplasmosis, blastomycosis, and histoplasmosis were performed. The toxoplasmosis IgM titer was positive so the llama was placed on sulfadimethoxine. When the symptoms worsened, the eye was removed and the tumor was discovered only on histopathologic examination of the globe.[41] In 2006 a case of a malignant nonteratoid medulloepithelioma was published.[42] This patient was a 6-year-old female llama that had tearing, buphthalmos, and a visible intraocular mass. The eye was removed but a mass appeared in the orbit 1 month later. Although radiation therapy initially shrunk the mass, it returned along with lymphadenopathy and masses in the mandible. The animal was killed and metastatic disease was seen in the orbit, mandible, mandibular lymph nodes, lungs, liver, and mesenteric and sublumbar lymph nodes. Histopathologic evaluation of all of the masses in the organs, lymph nodes, orbit, and globe was similar, and the diagnosis was a primary medulloepithelioma in the eye with systemic metastases.[42]

Another primitive tumor, a retinoblastoma, was found in the left eye of a pregnant, 6-year-old llama that was enucleated after the clinical signs of chronic epiphora, buphthalmos, and vision loss failed to respond to therapy.[43] Histopathologic results and results of immunohistochemical analysis showed that the tumor was a retinoblastoma.[43] In people retinoblastomas occur in children; they are often hereditary[44] and malignant. No metastases were reported in this llama and it was still alive 4 years after the eye was removed.

Two cases of intraocular melanomas in alpacas have been published. Hamor and colleagues reported a case of a 2-year-old alpaca with an intraocular melanoma that had been presented for a corneal opacity.[14] The opacity was edema caused by 2 large, pigmented iridial masses pressing on the cornea. Histopathologic examination showed that these were parts of the same melanoma. A 10-year-old pregnant female alpaca was presented to a veterinary clinic in New Zealand for evaluation of a discolored and enlarged right eye. The enucleated globe was firm and on sectioning for histopathologic examination a 5- by 6-mm piece of bone was found that was surrounded by a soft-tissue mass. Immunohistochemistry confirmed that the mass was a melanoma and that the neoplastic melanocytes were probably the progenitors of the bone.[45]

SUMMARY

Although the information about the ocular diseases to which camelids are susceptible is increasing, much still remains to be learned. In particular, genetic studies into the potential heritability and mode of inheritance of diseases such as congenital nasolacrimal diseases, cataracts, and colobomas may be valuable for camelid owners and veterinary practitioners advising them about breeding programs.

REFERENCES

1. Anderson DE, Whitehead CE. Preface. Vet Clin North Am Food Anim Pract 2009; 25:xi–xii.
2. Gionfriddo JR, Gionfriddo JP, Krohne SG. Ocular diseases of llamas: 194 cases (1980–1993). J Am Vet Med Assoc 1997;210:1784–7.
3. Duke ES. System of ophthalmology. In: The eye in evolution, vol. 1. St Louis (MO): CV Mosby; 1958. p. 458–70.
4. Sapienza JS, Isaza R, Johnson RD, et al. Anatomic and radiographic study of the lacrimal apparatus of llamas. Am J Vet Res 1992;53:1007–9.
5. Andrews SE, Willis AM, Anderson DE. Density of corneal endothelial cells, cornea thickness and corneal diameters in normal eyes of llamas and alpacas. Am J Vet Res 2002;63:326–9.
6. Webb AA, Cullen CL, Lamont LA. Brainstem auditory evoked responses and ophthalmic findings in llamas and alpacas in eastern Canada. Can Vet J 2006; 47:74–7.
7. Gelatt KN, Otzen Martinic GB, Flaneig JL, et al. Results of ophthalmic examinations of 29 alpacas. J Am Vet Med Assoc 1995;206:1204–7.
8. Willis AM, Mutti DO, Anderson DE, et al. Refractive error in llamas and alpacas. In: Proceedings 31st Annual Meeting Am Col Vet Ophthalmol, Montreal (QC), Canada: 2000. p. 26.
9. Gionfriddo JR. Ophthalmology. Vet Clin North Am Food Anim Pract 1994;16: 371–82.
10. Gionfriddo JR, Friedman DS. Ophthalmology of South American camelids: llamas, alpacas, guanacos, and vicuñas. In: Howard JL, editor. Current veterinary therapy: food animal practice. 3rd edition. Philadelphia: WB Saunders; 1993. p. 042–0.
11. Nuhsbaum MT, Gionfriddo JR, Powell CC, et al. Intraocular pressure in normal llamas (Lama glama) and alpacas (Lama pacos). Vet Ophthalmol 2000;3:31–4.
12. Mangan BG, Gionfriddo JR, Powell CC. Bilateral nasolacrimal duct atresia in a cria. Vet Ophthalmol 2008;11:49–54.
13. Gionfriddo JR, Blair M. Congenital cataracts and persistent hyaloid vasculature in a llama (Lama glama). Vet Ophthalmol 2002;5:65–70.
14. Hamor RE, Roberts SM, Severin GA. Intraocular melanoma in an alpaca. Vet Ophthalmol 1999;2:193–6.
15. Hendrix DV, Bochsler PN, Saladino B, et al. Malignant teratoid medulloepithelioma in a llama. Vet Pathol 2000;37:680–3.
16. Borkowski R, Moore PA, Mumford S, et al. Adaptations of a subpalpebral lavage system used for llamas (Lama glama) and a harbor seal (Phoca vitulina). J Zoo Wildl Med 2007;38:453–9.

17. Lavach JD. Large animal ophthalmology. St Louis (MO): Mosby–Year Book; 1990.
18. Schuh JCL, Ferguson JG, Fischer MA. Congenital coloboma in a llama. Can Vet J 1991;32:432–3.
19. Roberts SR. Congenital posterior ectasia of the sclera in the collie dog. Am J Ophthalmol 1960;50:451–5.
20. Sila GH, Morreale RJ, Lorimer DW, et al. A retrospective evaluation of the diamond burr superficial keratectomy in the treatment of spontaneous chronic corneal erosions in dogs from 2006 to 2008. Proceedings of the 40th Annual Conference of the American College of Veterinary Ophthalmologists. Chicago (IL), November 2009. p. 73.
21. Richter M, Grest P, Spiess B. Bilateral lipid keratopathy and atherosclerosis in an alpaca (*Lama pacos*) due to hypercholesterolemia. J Vet Intern Med 2008;20: 1503–7.
22. Rodriguez-Alvaro A, Fonzolez-Alonso-Alegre EM, Delclaux-Real del Asua M, et al. Surgical correction of a corneal perforation in an alpaca (*Lama pacos*). J Zoo Wildl Med 2005;36:336–9.
23. Barrie KP, Jacobson E, Peiffer RL Jr. Unilateral cataract with lens coloboma and bilateral corneal edema in a guanaco. J Am Vet Med Assoc 1978;173:1251–2.
24. Powell CC, Nuhsbaum TM, Gionfriddo JR. Aqueous misdirection and ciliary block (malignant) glaucoma after cataract removal in a llama. Vet Ophthalmol 2002;5: 99–101.
25. Brightman AH, McLaughlin SA, Brumley B. Keratoconjunctivitis in a llama. Vet Med Small Anim Clin 1981;76:1776–7.
26. Fowler M. Medicine and surgery of South American camelids. Ames (IA): State University Press; 1989.
27. Valentine BA, Martin JM. Prevalence of neoplasia in llamas and alpacas (Oregon State University, 2001–2006). J Vet Diagn Invest 2007;19:202–4.
28. McCaulery CT, Campbell GA, Cummings CA, et al. Ossifying fibroma in a llama. J Diagn Invest 2000;12:473–6.
29. Boer M, Schoon HA. Untersuchungen zu erblich bedingten Augen- und ZNS-Ver-danderungen in einer Zuchtgruppe von Vikunjas (*Lama vicugna*) im Zoologi-schen Garten Hanover. Verhandlungsbericht des Internationalen Symposiums über die Erkanungen der Zootier 1984;26:159–64 [in German].
30. Donaldson LL, Holland M, Koch SA. Atracurium as an adjunct to halothane-oxy-gen anesthesia in a llama undergoing intraocular surgery. Vet Surg 1992;21:76–9.
31. Ingram KA, Sigler RL. Cataract removal in a young llama. Proceedings of the Annual Meeting of the American Association of Zoo Veterinarians. Tampa (FL), October 23–27, 1983.
32. Middleton JR, Moody MM, Parish SM. Diabetes mellitus in an adult alpaca (*Lama pacos*). Vet Rec 2005;157:520–2.
33. Rebhun WC, Jenkins RC, et al. An epizootic of blindness and encephalitis asso-ciated with a herpes virus indistinguishable from equine herpesvirus I in a herd of alpacas and llamas. J Am Vet Med Assoc 1988;192:953–6.
34. Paulsen ME, Young S, Smith JA, et al. Bilateral chorioretinitis, centripetal optic neuritis, and encephalitis in a llama. J Am Vet Med Assoc 1989;194:1305–8.
35. House JA, Gregg DA, Lubroth J, et al. Experimental equine herpesvirus-1 infec-tion in llamas (*Lama glama*). J Vet Diagn Invest 1991;3:137–43.
36. Grahn BH, Cullen CL, Wolfer J. Diagnostic ophthalmology. Can Vet J 2001;42: 575–6.
37. Pickett JP, Moore CP, Beehler BA, et al. Bilateral chorioretinitis secondary to disseminated aspergillosis in an alpaca. J Am Vet Med Assoc 1985;187:1241–3.

38. Adams R, Garry FB. Gram-negative bacterial infection in neonatal New World camelids: six cases (1985–1991). J Am Vet Med Assoc 1992;201:1419–24.
39. Harrison TM, Dubielzig RR, Harrison TR, et al. Enrofloxacin-induced retinopathy in a guanaco (*Lama guanicoe*). J Zoo Wildl Med 2006;37:545–8.
40. Cullen CL, Grahn BH. Congenital glaucoma in a llama. Proceedings 28th Annual Meeting Am Col Vet Ophthalmol, Santa Fe (NM), 1997. p. 52.
41. Hendrix DV, Bochsler PN, Saladino B, et al. Malignant nonteratoid ocular medulloepithelioma in a llama (*Lama glama*). J Vet Diagn Invest 2006;18:499–503.
42. Schoeniger S, Donner LR, VanAlstine W. Malignant teratoid medulloepthelioma in a llama. Vet Pathol 2000;37:680–3.
43. Fugaro MN, Kiuple M, Montiani-Ferreira F, et al. Retinoblastoma in the eye of a llama (*Lama glama*). Vet Ophthalmol 2005;8:287–90.
44. Ellias WJ, Lopez MBS, Golden WL, et al. Trilateral retinoblastoma variant indicative of the relevance of the retinoblastoma tumor-suppressor pathway to medulloblastomas in humans. J Neurosurg 2001;95:871–8.
45. Hill FI, Hughes SM. Osteogenic intraocular melanoma in an alpaca (*Vicugna pacos*). J Vet Diagn Invest 2009;21:171–3.

Porcine Ophthalmology

Sheldon Middleton, MA, VetMB, MRCVS

KEYWORDS

- Pig eye • Porcine ophthalmology • Cataract
- Diprosopus piglet

As has been noted in the past,[1,2] porcine ophthalmology as a subject has received little attention. It has been suggested that general practitioners should contribute more to this area of the literature. As a general practitioner doing just that, the author confirms that although there appears to have been an increase in literature about the anatomy of the pig eye because of an expansion in its use as a model for research, there has been little written about the development of veterinary medicine in the area. This limited literature is probably because pigs are (usually) a farmed rather than pet species. Consequently, pigs do not live into old age and have neither the attention nor resources focused on them as individuals, which companion species may have.

There has been a surge of interest in the use of the pig eye as a model for research because of the ethical and economical restrictions of using other species (eg, primates). Pig eyes share many similarities with human eyes.[3–10] They are phylogenetically close to humans and have a holangiotic retinal vasculature, no tapetum, cone photoreceptors in the outer retina,[6] and similar scleral thickness.[7] Pig models have been developed for retinitis pigmentosa, glaucoma, and retinal detachment[6,11,12] and for studying transscleral drug delivery.[7]

The gross anatomy of the pig eye was thoroughly described by Prince and colleagues[10] and Diesem.[13] The anatomic descriptions in this article present updates and not necessarily a complete anatomic review of the porcine eye.

THE ORBIT

The many breeds of pig produce as many shapes of skull and therefore orbit. The orbit is open and continuous with the temporal fossa. The pig has a separation of between 80° and 120° (average 90°) between its orbital axes. However, the visual axes are divided by only 60° to 70°. The field of vision is probably 260° to 275°, with an estimated binocular field of 30° to 50° above the snout (**Fig. 1**).[10]

The author works in a mixed small animal and pig first opinion practice and has nothing to disclose.
Acorn House Veterinary Surgery, Linnet Way, Brickhill, Bedford, MK41 7HN, UK
E-mail address: sm@cantab.net

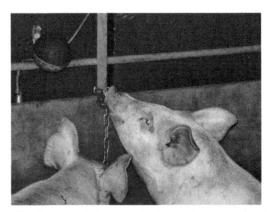

Fig. 1. Pig playing with a ball on a string as part of its environmental enrichment. This pig is demonstrating use of its estimated binocular field above the snout of 30° to 50°, allowing depth perception. (*Courtesy of* Dr M. Merrill PhD, Acorn House Veterinary Surgery, Bedford, UK.)

The frontal bone forms the roof and a portion of the medial wall of the orbit. The lacrimal bone completes the medial wall, and the zygomatic bone forms the ventral boundary. The temporal process of the zygomatic bone extends caudally ventral to the zygomatic process of the temporal bone. The inferior end of the orbital ligament attaches to the temporal process of the zygomatic bone. The orbit is completed by the attachment of the superior end of the orbital ligament to the zygomatic process of the frontal bone. The maxilla forms part of the rostral and rostroventral orbit. The wing of the presphenoid bone forms a large portion of the medial and caudal parts of the orbit. The wing of the basisphenoid bone forms a small part of the orbit. The ethmoid bone may appear in some porcine orbits below the frontal bone and above the palatine bone.

The orbit is conical. The extraocular muscles are anchored in a deep sphenoid fossa adjacent to the optic foramen. These muscle origins have a limited tendinous connection with each other but no true annulus of Zinn.[10]

The orbital venous sinus has been described as a site for obtaining blood samples in pigs weighing from 9 to 90 kg. The pig is placed in dorsal recumbency, and the fibrous conjunctival tissue is punctured using a glass pipette to rupture the venous sinus at the medial canthus just inside the nictitating membrane. This technique is difficult to carry out in the field and there are other preferred methods.[14]

THE GLOBE

The globe varies in dimensions because of the variation in size between breeds. McMenamin and Steptoe[9] found globe size to be 20.1 [0.74] × 23.5 [0.85] × 24.9 [0.87] (in mm [±SD]), using pigs of live weight greater than 90 kg and aged between 6 months and 2 years. The breed is not stated. Prince and colleagues[10] found the size to be 22–24 × 25 × 26–27 mm. No information on the animals used was given.

Intraocular pressure (IOP) (measured with an applanation tonometer [Tono-Pen XL; Medtronic, Jacksonville, FL, USA] under light general anesthesia [ketamine and xylazine]) is 15.2 mmHg (±1.8) in adult pigs (breed, age, and weight not stated).[6] Castejon and colleagues[15] found IOP to be 14.1 mmHg (±2.2) using a catheter inserted into the anterior chamber of the eye connected to a piezoelectric pressure sensor (Edwards

Lifesciences, Irvine, CA, USA), although the animal was under general anesthesia, using a constant rate infusion of propofol (Diprivan; AstraZeneca, Wilmington, DE, USA). These pigs weighed 20 kg, and the measurements were taken while in dorsal decubitus. Age and breed were not stated. The investigators found a linear relationship between blood pressure and IOP variations, using sodium nitroprusside and angiotensin II to pharmacologically vary blood pressure.

Rosolen and colleagues[16] found the IOP in minipigs using a Tono-Pen XL after topical application of oxybuprocaine to be 27.3 [3.45] (mmHg [±SD]) in the right eye and 26.3 [3.14] in the left eye. These were adult (15 months old) Göttingen minipigs and weighed between 13.8 and 17.8 kg. The pigs were awake and neither sedated nor anesthetized for the reading and were relaxed because familiar technicians were used. (Dr SG Rosolen, Moreau, France, personal communication, July 2010).

Cyclopia, anophthalmia, and microphthalmia have all been described as congenital abnormalities in Missouri piglets.[17] A hereditary microphthalmos has been described among the offspring of an American Yorkshire boar and concluded to be because of a dominant gene with low penetrance,[18] later considered to be inherited as an autosomal recessive trait.[19] Maternal vitamin A deficiency has been associated with anophthalmia, microphthalmia (most commonly), macrophthalmia, retinal dysplasia, and other ocular abnormalities, including blindness in piglets and adherence of eyelids to the cornea.[20] The gilts are usually normal. Deficiency in adults can also cause nyctalopia (night blindness) late in the disease. Affected adults may also show a head tilt, swaying gait, stiffness, and restlessness.[21–23]

A piglet was presented to the author's practice, which had 2 faces but 1 head and 1 body. The piglet was born alive and was able to use both mouths to feed. It was euthanised one day after birth. The piglet appeared externally to be triophthalmic (1 central eye shared by both faces and 2 lateral eyes, each associated with 1 face). The central eye had 1 set of eyelids. The (dead) piglet was imaged using magnetic resonance imaging and radiography. These tests revealed 2 central globes, occupying a shared orbit and eyelids. This type of conjoined twinning in swine has been noted before and described as diprosopus tetrophthalmos.[24] To the author's knowledge, no diprosopus piglets have been imaged in this way before (**Fig. 2**).

In a study, of the 112 observed Yucatan micropigs, hyaloid remnants and pupillary membrane remnants have been reported in 82.1% and 66.1%, respectively.[25]

The Cornea

The cornea is oval with the greater dimension being horizontal. The limbal conjunctiva is pigmented, contributing to a pigment ring bordering the cornea.[10] Corneal measurements can be found in **Table 1**. The normal porcine corneal epithelium contains angiostatin (an inhibitor of angiogenesis, which reduces retinal and corneal neovascularization) but not integrin $\alpha v \beta 3$ (a promoter of angiogenesis). The regulation of angiogenesis is an important factor in maintaining optical clarity.[26] Recent work has also indicated that the porcine cornea has almost isotropic mechanical behavior across different anatomic directions. Other species have different alignments of corneal stromal fibrils, resulting in anisotropic mechanical behavior, which is assumed to be because of the insertion of the rectus muscles and the need to resist distortion during eye movement.[27] It is not postulated as to why the porcine cornea displays this behavior; although the origin of the pig's extraocular muscles are unusually powerful, perhaps necessitating corneal mechanical isotropy (**Fig. 3**).

The porcine cornea consists of a surface epithelium, Bowman membrane (not easy to distinguish in the pig), substantia propria, Descemet membrane, and the endothelial layer.[13]

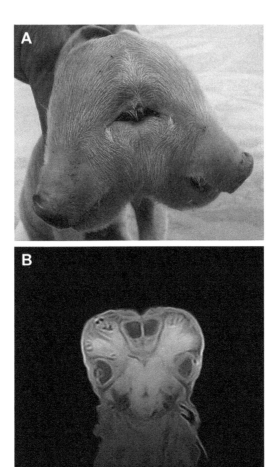

Fig. 2. (*A*) Two-faced (diprosopus) piglet. The piglet was born alive but was later eutha-nized. Note the single pair of central eyelids. (*B*) Magnetic resonance image of the same piglet (taken postmortem), showing 4 globes present in total (tetrophthalmos). The two most rostral globes share a single set of eyelids. (*Courtesy of* D. J. Chennells MRCVS, Acorn House Veterinary Surgery, Bedford, UK [*A*]; and the Radiology Department, Department of Veterinary Medicine, University of Cambridge, Cambridge, UK, with permission [*B*].)

The Lens

The lens has a steeper posterior curvature and in this respect is similar to that in man. The capsule varies between 5 to 30 μm in thickness.[10]

Congenital cataracts (posterior cortical pinpoint opacities) have been reported in 20.5% of observed Yucatan micropigs aged between 7 and 12 months.[25] The author has seen a Duroc boar, which has had congenital cataracts from birth. It is now 3 years old. An ocular searching nystagmus was present at all times with no distinct fast phase. The boar had learned to navigate using other senses. There was a slight pupil-lary light reflex in both eyes, but thorough examination of the eye was difficult. The dam of this boar was unlikely to have been fed an incomplete diet during gestation because she came from a commercial pig farm. Two offspring of the boar were recently reported by the farmer as having cataracts (**Fig. 4**).

Some bilateral cortical opacities in mature sows have been attributed to hygromycin B, an aminoglycoside antibiotic used to control gastrointestinal helminths. The cataracts begin as central, posterior, subcapsular opacities and then progress to complete, dense, cortical, often asymmetrical, cataracts. Microscopically, the cataractous lenses consisted of swollen lens fibers and subcapsular vacuolation. Cataract formation due to added hygromycin B in the ration of pigs appears to be dose dependent and possibly cumulative.[28–31] Norton[32] reported an outbreak of cataracts in sows being fed hygromycin B but was unable to attribute the cataract formation to the feed.

Yucatan minipig sows fed with alloxan (a glucose analogue) gave birth to piglets with nuclear cataracts. The cataracts did not progress or significantly affect vision.[2]

Cataract formation may be associated with niacin or riboflavin deficiency.[33] Cataracts in 35-day-old piglets that were fed a diet artificially low in riboflavin were noted to be located posterior to the equator and manifested by a swelling and separation of the lens fibers. Ballooning of the columnar cells of the basal layer of the corneal epithelium was observed.[34]

The Iris, Ciliary Body, and Choroid

McMenamin and Steptoe[9] made the following observations about the porcine ciliary body. As in most nonprimates, the ciliary body is split into 2 portions (stromal and scleral) by the ciliary cleft. The anterior portion of the stromal part of the ciliary body consists of characteristic radially arranged ciliary processes (95 main ciliary processes with a smaller process between each pair of larger ones[10]). The scleral portion of the ciliary body consists of a few bands of ciliary smooth muscle fibers embedded in irregular connective tissue close to the sclera. The ciliary muscle in all areas contains an anterior portion of circumferentially oriented bundles and a posterior portion in which the fibers have a longitudinal orientation.[9] The ciliary muscle shows clear regional differences throughout the circumference of the anterior eye, and it has been postulated that this muscle may be acting to regulate the elastic forces in the choroid rather than as an accommodative muscle.[35]

The ciliary cleft (an extension of the anterior chamber) extends approximately 1.5 mm into the ciliary body and is 0.3 to 0.4 mm at its widest point. The cleft is crossed by stout pectinate ligaments and delicate uveal cords. The corneoscleral meshwork (analogous to the cribriform layer of primates) and the angular aqueous plexus (a series of collector vessels analogous to the primate canal of Schlemm) are housed in a distinct internal scleral sulcus. The corneoscleral meshwork is comparable in size to the human trabecular meshwork.[9]

The strands of the porcine pectinate ligament are short (radial length <0.5 mm[36]), slender (50–60 μm in thickness[9]), and slightly pigmented. The intertrabecular spaces are round or oval, giving a characteristic cribriform appearance.

The pupil of the pig is slightly horizontally oval, becoming circular when dilated. There is considerable pigment on the anterior surface of the iris and no corpora nigra.[10]

Heterochromia iridis has an estimated incidence of 5% to 7% in swine. The condition has been described in miniature swine and shows an autosomal recessive inheritance pattern. It appears unrelated to coat color in some species but closely related to white coats in the American Yorkshire pigs (related to the Large White in the United Kingdom). Histology shows reduced pigmentation of the iridal stroma.[37]

The pig, unlike other domestic animals, has no tapetum, which is seen as an advantage for certain types of research because imaging of the posterior pole is easier.[7] The

Table 1
Measurement of anatomic parameters of the eye of pigs

Parameter	Measurement	Notes	References
Globe Size (mm) [±SD]	20.1 [0.74] × 23.5 [0.85] × 24.9 [0.87] 22–24 × 25 × 26–27		9,a 10,b
Globe Volume (ml) [±SD]	6.5 [0.3]		9
Anterior Chamber Volume (ml)	300		9
Number of Ciliary Processes	95 main processes	Smaller processes between each pair of larger ones	10
Ciliary Cleft Depth (mm)	1.5		9
Ciliary Cleft Width (mm)	0.3–0.4 at widest point		9
Pectinate Ligament Radial Length (mm)	<0.5		36
Pectinate Ligament Width (μm)	50–60		9
Intraocular pressure (mm Hg) [±SD]	15.2 [SEM 1.8] 14.1 [2.2] 27.3 [3.45] OD 26.3 [3.14] OS	Data from anesthetized animals Data from anesthetized animals Data from minipigs (not anesthetized)	6,c 15,d 16,e
Scleral thickness near the limbus (point of maximum thickness) (mm) [±SD]	0.83 [0.20], small pigs 0.91 [0.17], medium pigs 1.12 [0.23], large pigs^f 0.55		7 10
Scleral thickness at the point of minimum thickness (mm) [±SD]	0.31 [0.07], small pigs 0.35 [0.1], medium pigs 0.43 [0.16], large pigs	5 mm (small and medium-sized pigs) and 6mm (large pigs) from limbus	7
Scleral thickness at the equator (mm) [±SD]	0.56 [0.11], small pigs 0.73 [0.14], medium pigs 0.86 [0.18], large pigs 0.25		7 10

		Reference
Mean scleral surface area (cm^2) [±SD]	7.78 [0.66], small pigs	7
	9.66 [0.75], medium pigs	
	11.92 [1.57], large pigs	
Mean corneal surface area (cm^2) [±SD]	1.09 [0.07], small pigs	7
	1.15 [0.09], medium pigs	
	1.4 [0.19], large pigs	
Corneal dimensions (mm)	17–19 × 14–16.5	10
	14–16 × 13–14	13
Corneal thickness (mm)	<1	10
Optic nerve head dimensions (mm)	4.0–4.5 × 2.0–2.5	42,g
Retinal cone density (per mm^2)	19,000–24,000 (maximum)	42
	39,000 (maximum)	4,h
	16,400 (mean)	
Total photoreceptor density (per mm^2)	200,000 (maximum)	4
	138,500 (mean)	

Abbreviations: OD, oculus dexter; OS, oculus sinister; SEM, standard error of the mean.

[a] From pigs heavier than 90 kg live weight aged between 6 months and 2 years, breed not stated.
[b] No information given on animals used.
[c] Results obtained with an applanation tonometer under light general anesthesia (ketamine and xylazine).
[d] Results obtained using a catheter inserted into the anterior chamber of the eye connected to a piezoelectric pressure sensor while the animal was under general anesthesia, using a constant rate infusion of propofol.
[e] Results obtained from Göttingen minipigs using an applanation tonometer after application of oxybuprocaine.
[f] Small pigs (≤8 kg, n = 38); medium pigs (8.1–26.9 kg, n = 40); large pigs (≥27 kg, n = 42).
[g] From adult pigs aged 3 to 5 years.
[h] From pigs aged 8 to 12 months.

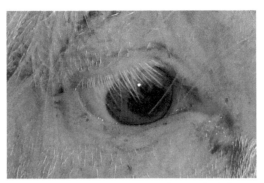

Fig. 3. Close-up of the external features of a young (2 month old) pig's eye (OD). Note the ring of conjunctival pigmentation contributing to the pigment ring bordering the cornea. Long cilia are present on the upper lid only.

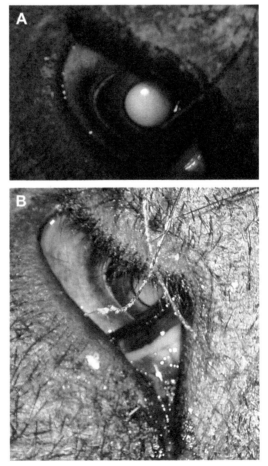

Fig. 4. (*A, B*) Two views of the same eye (OD) of a Duroc boar with congenital cataracts. The poor quality of photography reflects the difficulty in examining and restraining large pigs.

porcine choroid varies in thickness with a prominent Bruch membrane between the choroid and retina.[13]

A strain of the miniature Sinclair swine has been described, which has a high incidence (54%) of cutaneous malignant melanomas at birth, rising to 85% of the population at the age of 1 year because previously tumor-free animals developed tumors. No intraocular melanomas were found. The tumors usually spontaneously regress, but the regression was often accompanied by depigmentation of the skin, hair, and eyes. The regression initiated a uveitis and depigmentation of the uveal tract because of immune-mediated destruction of normal melanocytes by macrophages. Secondary ocular changes often led to blindness. It is likely that the same immune response was responsible for the tumor regression.[38] Recent work has concluded that the regression is associated with a loss of telomerase activity and reduction of telomeric repeats in the melanoma, leading to cell death.[39]

The Sclera

The porcine sclera can be highly pigmented, particularly in those breeds with dark hair coats.[10,13] The thickness varies across the globe, with the thickest point at the corneal scleral limbus (see **Table 1**). The thinnest area as noted by Prince and colleagues[10] was at the equator, but recent work[7] has shown this to be 5 to 6 mm posterior to the limbus. The total surface area of the sclera has also been measured (see **Table 1**). The measurements are found to be close to those of humans.

The porcine lamina cribrosa has a pigmented linear fascial groove when viewed in cross section. The groove has not been reported in other species, which may be a vestige of the embryonic optic fissure.[40]

The Retina

The pig retina is relatively mature at birth with all layers and retinal cell types present in 1-week-old animals with some degree of retinal maturation occurring during the postnatal period.[3] The porcine retina is similar to that of man. One of the most easily observable features is an oval optic nerve head. The fundus color varies from red-brown to gray, and there is no tapetum, as previously mentioned. There are many cones in the retina, suggesting a diurnal evolutionary history.[10] Photoreceptor cell distribution has regional differences in the porcine retina, with the overall ratio of rods to cones being 7–8:1.[4,41,42] There is a streak of high cone density situated parallel to the horizontal axis whose center corresponds with an area close to the posterior pole, which is sufficiently free of blood vessels to suggest a macular area or area centralis.[4,10,42] This region is expected to be more sensitive to color and high acuity vision, similar to the fovea of humans.[4] A second area of high cone density has been described in the nasal midperiphery by Gerke and colleagues[42] but not by Chandler and colleagues.[4] The thickness of the retinal layers corresponds closely with the human retina.[41]

There is no central retinal artery and vein in pigs. The retinal circulation is holangiotic and major vessels lie superficially within the retina, radiating from the optic disk either centrally or near its borders. There are 4 major retinal arteries deriving from the main ciliary artery of the orbit, which is in turn derived from the external carotid circulation via the external ophthalmic artery. Ultimately, these vessels branch to form an extensive vascular tree over the retina. There are 2 to 4 layers of capillaries arising from the retinal arterioles. Again, overall, the structure of the retinal vasculature of the pig is similar to that of the human (**Fig. 5**).[10,43–45]

Arsanilic acid is one of the several organic arsenicals, which has been used therapeutically for swine dysentery and as a growth stimulant in some areas. Excessive

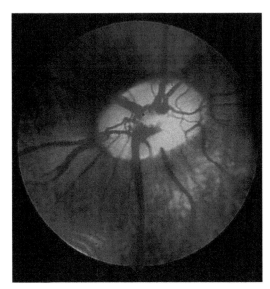

Fig. 5. Normal fundus of a minipig. Note the holangiotic retinal circulation and major vessels lying superficially within the retina, radiating from the optic disk either (as in this case) centrally or near its borders. The porcine fundus does not have a tapetal zone. (*Courtesy of* S. G. Rosolen PhD, Centre de Recherche, Institut de la Vision, Moreau, France.)

intake, long-term administration, or normal intake with restricted water intake can cause clinical signs of blindness and pupillary dilation, torticollis, weakness, and inco-ordination. Pupillary light reflexes are absent and bilateral optic disk atrophy is present, characterized by pallor, well-defined margins, and narrowed retinal arterioles[33,46–49]

Developing pigs that were fed a low-zinc diet showed an exaggerated number of cone nuclei displaced towards the retinal pigment epithelium. The overall size of the retinal pigment epithelium was larger in pigs fed a low-zinc diet than in those fed a controlled diet. The study suggests a role for zinc in cytoprotection and metabolic homeostasis during photoreception.[50]

ACCESSORY OCULAR ORGANS

The lacrimal gland of the pig is relatively small and thin and is situated laterodorsally to the globe. It is roughly triangular and serous in form. The pig has both a lacrimal and harderian gland. The harderian gland is situated infralaterally within the orbit, discharging via ducts onto the bulbar surface of the nictitating membrane and the conjunctival sac. The nictitans gland is large and active and discharges mostly mucous secretions through many ducts into the conjunctival sac. The nictitating membrane covers the cartilage of the third eyelid and is intimately associated with the nictitating gland, which lies on the palpebral side of the cartilage.[10,13]

The secretions drain via the lacrimal system. There are dorsal and ventral lacrimal ducts but the ventral duct is usually nonfunctional. The 2 ducts meet without forming a dilatation. There is no lacrimal sac in the pig.[13]

The eyelids of the pig have limited movement. The pig blinks approximately 10 times per minute, with 90% of the blinks being bilateral.[51] There is considerable fat under the skin, producing a deep palpebral fold in the upper eyelid a few millimeters from the lid margin. Long, coarse cilia are present on the upper lid only (see **Fig. 3**). There is no palpebral fold on the lower lid. The equivalent of the human tarsal plate is a sheet of connective tissue surrounding the meibomian gland. This sheet extends from the lid margin upwards but has little effect on lid rigidity. The main glands in the pig's eye are large, numerous, modified sweat glands rather than meibomian glands as in other species. These glands lie between the muscle bundles of the extensive orbicularis muscle. There are numerous goblet cells in the conjunctiva of the lids.[10,13]

The potbellied pig has a large amount of subcutaneous fat in the forehead and periocular region, which contributes to the development of entropion. This fat can sometimes hypertrophy and cause impaired eyelid opening, if not entropion, requiring surgical correction. Surgical correction of this problem has been reported using the Stades technique,[52] modified Hotz-Celsus technique, and excision of the redundant fat and skin. A modified brow sling technique may be effective.[2,53–55]

Chlamydiae were isolated from conjunctival swabs from pigs with a combination of conjunctivitis and keratoconjunctivitis, with or without mucopurulent rhinitis. It has not been established whether these were resident microflora or pathogens, although it has been suggested that chlamydiae play a role in conjunctivitis and keratoconjunctivitis in swine. It may be difficult to isolate chlamydiae from conjunctival swabs. *Mycoplasma* is also likely to play a role in the pathogenesis of some cases of conjunctivitis and keratoconjunctivitis.[56] *Mycoplasma* sp, streptococci, and coagulase-negative staphylococci as well as *Mycoplasma*-like organisms were isolated from pigs with varying degrees of lacrimation, conjunctival hyperemia, chemosis, and mucopurulent conjunctivitis.[57] A pathogenic interplay between porcine Circovirus type 2, causing clinical disease (postweaning multisystemic wasting syndrome) in weaned piglets, and chlamydial species (*Chlamydophila abortus* and *Chlamydophila suis*), causing clinical disease (conjunctival and reproductive failure) in boars, sows, and gilts, has been suggested.[58]

Eyelid swelling is seen in edema disease (*Escherichia coli* infection) and commonly affects recently weaned pigs in good condition.[59]

Conjunctivitis can be seen in pigs affected by swine influenza, usually associated with sudden onset respiratory disease, pyrexia, and anorexia. Morbidity approaches 100%.[60]

Ophthalmia neonatorum can be seen in piglets.[23]

The most common cause of lacrimation in swine is ammonia at concentrations higher than 25 ppm. Humans can detect ammonia at 10 ppm, so a diagnosis can easily be made by sniffing the environment and moving the pig to a clean air area where the signs should subside.[33]

Ocular Manifestations of Systemic Disease

Pseudorabies (Aujeszky disease) is caused by an α-herpesvirus. Outbreaks are characterized by blindness, depression, head pressing, and death. Death or recovery usually occurs by day 3 but those that survive are usually permanently blind.[61] Corneal ulceration and keratoconjunctivitis with persistent opacities have been observed in experimentally inoculated porcine corneas. Transient iritis also developed.[62]

Classical swine fever is caused by a Pestivirus in the Flaviviridae group. The fever occurs in several forms, including acute, subacute, chronic, and persistent. Conjunctivitis is frequent in the acute form, with copious ocular discharge and periocular crusting. Iridociliary congestion, edema, anterior uveitis, focal choroiditis, retinitis, and optic neuritis may also occur with time (**Fig. 6**).[63]

African swine fever is caused by the African swine fever virus of Asfarviridae. This fever is a highly lethal hemorrhagic disease, with mortality rates approaching

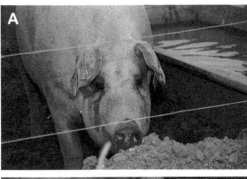

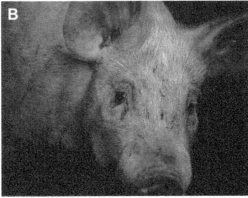

Fig. 6. (*A*) Pig with classical swine fever showing copious ocular discharge. (*B*) Pig with classical swine fever showing conjunctivitis in OD. (*Courtesy of* JD Mackinnon FRCVS, Pig Health and Production Consultancy, Saxmundham, UK.)

100%.[64] Blindness with phthisis bulbi has been reported along with conjunctival hemorrhages early in the febrile stage of the disease. Serous to mucopurulent conjunctival and nasal discharges may be present later in the disease course.[1] There is an element of conjunctival excretion of the virus, generally after the onset of pyrexia.[65]

Swine are the natural intermediate host of *Taenia solium*, and previously humans were thought to be the sole definitive hosts, whereupon the tapeworm would cause cysticercosis in both pig and man. Recently, an alternative pig-to-pig route of transmission has been reported.[66] The larval stage of *T solium* (known as *Cysticercus cellulosae)* may invade the eye. Both orbital and intraocular cysts have been reported. A severe granulomatous endophthalmitis or panophthalmitis is usually found once the cysticercus has been dead for some time, with most investigators believing that no inflammatory exudate is found while the parasite is alive.[67]

Porcine paramyxovirus is a viral infectious disease characterized by encephalitis, corneal opacity (arising from edema and giving rise to the name blue eye disease), pneumonia in young pigs, and reproductive failure in sows. The main features in piglets aged 2 to 21 days are central nervous system manifestations and corneal opacity. Older pigs seem to be more resistant, and only corneal opacity is commonly observed.[68] Affected pigs may develop conjunctivitis with epiphora, chemosis, swollen eyelids, and ocular discharge adherent to the eyelids. Vesicle formation, ulcers and keratoconus have been observed in the cornea. Microscopic changes in the eye are infiltration of the iridocorneal endothelium, corneoscleral angle, and cornea of neutrophils, macrophages, or mononuclear cells. The external sheet of the cornea often has cytoplasmic vesicles. Diagnosis is based on virus isolation and clinical signs, and there is no specific therapy at present.[69,70]

REFERENCES

1. Vestre WA. Porcine ophthalmology. Vet Clin North Am Large Anim Pract 1984;6: 667–76.
2. Townsend WM. Food and fiber-producing animal ophthalmology. In: Gelatt KN, editor. Veterinary ophthalmology. 4th edition. Ames (IA): Blackwell Publishing; 2007. p. 1275–335.
3. Guduric-Fuchs J, Ringland LJ, Gu P, et al. Immunohistochemical study of pig retinal development. Mol Vis 2009;15:1915–28.
4. Chandler MJ, Smith PJ, Samuelson DA, et al. Photoreceptor density of the domestic pig retina. Vet Ophthalmol 1999;2:179–84.
5. Kivell TL, Doyle SK, Madden RH, et al. An interactive method for teaching anatomy of the human eye for medical students in ophthalmology clinical rotations. Anat Sci Educ 2009;2:173–8.
6. Ruiz-Ederra J, Garcia M, Hernandez M, et al. The pig eye as a novel model of glaucoma. Exp Eye Res 2005;81:561–9.
7. Olsen TW, Sanderson S, Feng X, et al. Porcine sclera: thickness and surface area. Invest Ophthalmol Vis Sci 2002;43(8):2529–32.
8. Humphray S, Scott C, Clark R, et al. A high utility integrated map of the pig genome. Genome Biol 2007;8(7):R139.
9. McMenamin PG, Steptoe RJ. Normal anatomy of the aqueous humour outflow system in the domestic pig eye. J Anat 1991;178:65–77.
10. Prince JH, Diesem DC, Eglitis I, et al. The pig. In: Anatomy and histology of the eye and orbit in domestic animals. Springfield (IL): Charles C Thomas; 1960. p. 210–33.
11. Petters RM, Alexander CA, Wells KD, et al. Genetically engineered large animal model for studying cone photoreceptor survival and degeneration in retinitis pigmentosa. Nat Biotechnol 1997;15:965–70.
12. Iandiev I, Uckermann O, Pannicke T, et al. Glial cell reactivity in a porcine model of retinal detachment. Invest Ophthalmol Vis Sci 2006;47:2161–71.
13. Diesem CD. Porcine sense organs and common integument. In: Getty R, editor. Sisson and Grossman's the anatomy of the domestic animals. Philadelphia: Saunders; 1975. p. 1409–17.
14. Muirhead MR. Blood sampling in pigs. In Pract 1981;3:16–20.
15. Castejon H, Chiquet C, Savy O, et al. Effect of acute increase in blood pressure on intraocular pressure in pigs and humans. Invest Ophthalmol Vis Sci 2010; 51(3):1599–605.
16. Rosolen SG, Rigaudière F, Le Gargasson J-F. [Un nouveau modèle d'hyperpression oculaire induite chez le miniporc]. Journal Français d'Ophtalmologie 2003; 26(3):259–67 [in French].
17. Selby LA, Hopps HC, Edmonds LD. Comparative aspects of congenital malformations in man and swine. J Am Vet Med Assoc 1971;159:1485–90.
18. Roberts LD. Microphthalmia in swine. J Hered 1948;39:146–8.
19. Howard J, Smith R. Current veterinary therapy 4: food animal practice. 4th edition. Philadelphia: WB Saunders; 1999.
20. Palludan B. The teratogenic effect of vitamin A deficiency in pigs. Acta Vet Scand 1961;2:32–59.

21. Watt JA, Barlow RM. Microphthalmia in piglets with avitaminosis a as the probable cause. Vet Rec 1956;68:780–3.

22. Hale F. Pigs born without eyeballs. J Hered 1933;24:105–6.

23. Slatter DH. Fundamentals of veterinary ophthalmology. 3rd edition. Philadelphia: W B Saunders Company; 2001.

24. Selby LA, Khalili A, Stewart RW, et al. Pathology and epidemiology of conjoined twinning in swine. Teratology 1973;8:1–10.

25. Saint-Macary G, Berthoux C. Ophthalmic observations in the young Yucatan micropig. Lab Anim Sci 1994;44:334–7.

26. Pearce JW, Janardhan KS, Caldwell S, et al. Angiostatin and integrin αvβ3 in the feline, bovine, canine, equine, porcine and murine retina and cornea. Vet Ophthalmol 2007;10(5):313–9.

27. Elsheikh A, Alhasso D. Mechanical anisotropy of porcine cornea and correlation with stromal microstructure. Exp Eye Res 2009;88:1084–91.

28. Sanford SE, Dukes TW. Acquired bilateral cortical cataracts in mature sows. J Am Vet Med Assoc 1978;173:852–3.

29. Sanford SE, Dukes TW, Creighton MO, et al. Cortical cataracts induced by hygromycin B in swine. Am J Vet Res 1981;42:1534–7.

30. Creighton MO, Trevithick JR, Sanford SE, et al. Modeling cortical cataractogenesis. IV. Induction by hygromycin B in vivo (swine) and in vitro (rat lens). Exp Eye Res 1982;34:467–76.

31. Cargill CF, Giesecke PR, Heap PA, et al. Bilateral cortical cataracts in sows. Aust Vet J 1983;60(10):312–3.

32. Norton JH. Cataracts in sows. Aust Vet J 1980;56:403.

33. Straw BE, Dewey CE, Wilson MR. Differential diagnosis of swine diseases. In: Straw BE, D'Allaire S, Mengeling WL, et al, editors. Diseases of swine. 8th edition. Ames (IA): Iowa State University Press/Blackwell Science Ltd; 1999. p. 41–86.

34. Miller ER, Johnston RL, Hoefer JA, et al. The riboflavin requirement of the baby pig. J Nutr 1954;52:405–13.

35. May CA, Skorski LM, Lutjen-Drecoll E. Innervation of the porcine ciliary muscle and outflow region. J Anat 2005;206:231–6.

36. Simoens P, De Geest J, Lauwers H. Comparative morphology of the pectinate ligaments of domestic mammals, as observed under the dissecting microscope and the scanning electron microscope. J Vet Med Sci 1996;58:977–82.

37. Gelatt KN, Rempel WE, Makambera TP, et al. Heterochromia irides in miniature swine. J Hered 1973;64:343–7.

38. Feeney-Burns L, Burns RP, Gao C. Ocular pathology in melanomatous Sinclair miniature swine. Am J Pathol 1988;131:62–72.

39. Pathak S, Multani AS, McConkey DJ, et al. Spontaneous regression of cutaneous melanoma in Sinclair swine is associated with defective telomerase activity and extensive telomere erosion. Int J Oncol 2000;17(6):1219–24.

40. Brooks DE, Arellano E, Kubilis PS, et al. Histomorphometry of the porcine scleral lamina cribrosa surface. Vet Ophthalmol 1998;1:129–35.

41. Beauchemin ML. The fine structure of the pig's retina. Albrecht Von Graefes Arch Clin Exp Ophthalmol 1974;190:27–45.

42. Gerke CG Jr, Hao Y, Wong F. Topography of rods and cones in the retina of the domestic pig. Hong Kong Med J 1995;1:302–8.

43. Bloodworth JM Jr, Gutgesell HP Jr, Engerman RL. Retinal vasculature of the pig. Light and electron microscope studies. Exp Eye Res 1965;4:174–8.

44. Rootman J. Vascular system of the optic nerve head and retina in the pig. Br J Ophthalmol 1971;55:808–19.

45. Simoens P, De Schaepdrijver L, Lauwers H. Morphologic and clinical study of the retinal circulation in the miniature pig. A morphology of the retinal microvasculature. Exp Eye Res 1992;54:965–73.
46. Witzel DA, Smith EL, Beerwinkle KR, et al. Arsanilic acid-induced blindness in swine: electroretinographic and visually evoked responses. Am J Vet Res 1976; 37(5):521–4.
47. Menges RW, Kintner LD, Selby LA, et al. Arsanilic acid blindness in pigs. Vet Med Small Anim Clin 1970;65:565–8.
48. Vorhies MW, Sleight SD, Whitehair CK. Toxicity of arsanilic acid in swine as influenced by water intake. Cornell Vet 1969;59:3–9.
49. Oliver WT, Roe CK. Arsanilic acid poisoning in swine. J Am Vet Med Assoc 1957; 130:177–8.
50. Samuelson DA, Swank A, Whitley RD, et al. Morphological and morphometric effects of low-zinc diet on the young porcine eye. Progress in Veterinary and Comparative Ophthalmology 1992;3(2):58–66.
51. Gum GG, Gelatt KN, Esson DW. Physiology of the eye. In: Gelatt KN, editor. Veterinary ophthalmology, 4th edition, vol. 1. Ames (IA): Blackwell Publishing; 2007. p. 149–82.
52. Stades FC. A new method for surgical correction of upper eyelid trichiasis-entropion: operation method. J Am Anim Hosp Assoc 1987;23:603–6.
53. Allbaugh RA, Davidson HJ. Surgical correction of periocular fat pads and entropion in a potbellied pig (Sus scrofa). Vet Ophthalmol 2009;12(2):115–8.
54. Andrea CR, George LW. Surgical correction of periocular fat pad hypertrophy in pot-bellied pigs. Vet Surg 1999;28:311–4.
55. Linton LL, Collins BK. Entropion repair in a Vietnamese pot-bellied pig. J Small Exotic Anim Med 1993;2:124–7.
56. Rogers DG, Andersen AA, Hogg A, et al. Conjunctivitis and keratoconjunctivitis associated with chlamydiae in swine. J Am Vet Med Assoc 1993;203:1321–3.
57. Rogers DG, Frey ML, Hogg A. Conjunctivitis associated with a Mycoplasma-like organism in swine. J Am Vet Med Assoc 1991;198(3):450–2.
58. Schautteet K, Beeckman DS, Delava P, et al. Possible pathogenic interplay between Chlamydia suis, Chlamydophila abortus and PCV-2 on a pig production farm. Vet Rec 2010;166:329–33.
59. Gyles CL, Henton MM. Escherichia coli infections. In: Coetzer JA, Tustin RC, editors. Infectious diseases of livestock, 2nd edition, vol. 3. Cape Town (South Africa): Oxford University Press; 2004. p. 1560–77.
60. Thomson GR, Easterday BC. Swine influenza. In: Coetzer JA, Tustin RC, editors. Infectious diseases of livestock, 2nd edition, vol. 2. Cape Town (South Africa): Oxford University Press; 2004. p. 775–8.
61. Howarth JA, De Paoli A. An enzootic of pseudorabies in swine in California. J Am Vet Med Assoc 1968;152:1114–8.
62. Schneider WJ, Howarth JA. Clinical course and histopathalogic features of pseudorabies virus-induced keratoconjunctivitis in pigs. Am J Vet Res 1973;34: 393–401.
63. Saunders LZ, Jubb KV, Jones LD. The intraocular lesions of hog cholera. J Comp Pathol 1958;68:375–9.
64. Zsak L, Borca MV, Risatti GR, et al. Preclinical diagnosis of African swine fever in contact-exposed swine by a real-time PCR assay. J Clin Microbiol 2005;43: 112–9.
65. Greig A, Plowright W. The excretion of two virulent strains of African swine fever virus by domestic pigs. J Hyg 1970;68(4):673–82.

66. Gonzalez AE, Lopez-Urbina T, Tsang B, et al. Transmission dynamics of *Taenia solium* and potential for pig-to-pig transmission. Parasitol Int 2006;55:S131–5.
67. Cardenas-Ramierez L, Celis-Salgado P, Hernandez-Jauregui P. Ocular and orbital cysticercosis in hogs. Vet Pathol 1984;21:164–7.
68. Stephan HA, Gay GM, Ramirez TC. Encephalomyelitis, reproductive failure and corneal opacity (blue eye) in pigs, associated with a paramyxovirus infection. Vet Rec 1988;122:6–10.
69. Stephano AH. Blue eye disease. In: Straw BE, D'Allaire S, Mengeling WL, et al, editors. Diseases of swine. 8th edition;. Ames (IA): Iowa State university/Blackwell Science Ltd; 1999. p. 103–12.
70. Corona E. Porcine paramyxovirus (blue eye disease). The Pig Journal 2000;45: 115–8.

Postscript

The following article is an addition to Bovine Respiratory Disease, the July 2010 issue of Veterinary Clinics of North America: Food Animal Practice (Volume 26, Issue 2).

Bovine Parainfluenza-3 Virus

John A. Ellis, DVM, PhD

KEYWORDS

- Bovine parainfluenza-3 virus • Parainfluenza • Paramyxovirus
- Enzootic pneumonia • Bovine respiratory disease complex

HISTORICAL PERSPECTIVE

Bovine parainfluenza-3 virus (bPI$_3$V) was first isolated in the United States by workers at the US Department of Agriculture laboratory in Beltsville, Maryland, from the nasal discharge of cattle with shipping fever, and initially called myxovirus SF-4[1] in the August 1, 1959 issue of the *Journal of the American Veterinary Medical Association*. In the same issue, other workers at the University of Illinois, together with collaborators at the National Institutes of Health in Bethesda, Maryland, reported[2] on the apparent second isolation of the virus, and gave it its current name based on serologic relationships with the HA-1 strain of human parainfluenza or human parainfluenza-3 virus (hPI$_3$V)[3] in the then newly designated parainfluenza virus group.[4] Based on growth in the same cultured cells, ability to agglutinate erythrocytes from the same species, and essentially identical patterns of hemagglutination inhibition (HI) and virus neutralization (VN) activities by hyperimmune rabbit and chicken sera raised against the respective viruses, it was proposed that these 2 viruses were different strains of the same viral species, although, based on preliminary unpublished experiments, it was mentioned that "cattle may be relatively insusceptible to infection with the human strain."[3]

In the 1960s, growth characteristics, including differences among isolates, were described in detail. During this period and thereafter, bPI$_3$V was found to be endemic in cattle populations worldwide. In the 1970s and 1980s most of the seminal work on the pathogenesis of bPI$_3$V infections, documentation of interisolate genetic and antigenic differences, as well as the development and testing of parenteral and intranasal vaccines were completed. There have been few published studies on bPI$_3$V in the last 20 years. Work on bPI$_3$V since the last review of the agent in the *Veterinary Clinics of North America* in 1997[5] has focused on the viral variation and the possibility of cross-species transmission. Because of its endemicity, inclusion in commonly used combination vaccines, and the common failure to pursue or obtain specific etiologic diagnoses in field cases of respiratory disease, it has become a forgotten virus,

Department of Veterinary Microbiology, Western College of Veterinary Medicine, University of Saskatchewan, 52 Campus Drive, Saskatoon, Saskatchewan, S7N 5B4, Canada
E-mail address: john.ellis@usask.ca

Vet Clin Food Anim 26 (2010) 575–593
doi:10.1016/j.cvfa.2010.08.002
0749-0720/10/$ – see front matter © 2010 Elsevier Inc. All rights reserved.

much like its human counterpart, hPI$_3$V, which continues to a major clinical infection in infancy and childhood.[6] One purpose of this review is to emphasize that relegation to this status is unwarranted.

VIRUS CHARACTERISTICS

bPI$_3$V is in the genus Respirovirus of the subfamily Paramyxovirinae, order Mononega-virales, of the family Paramyxoviridae. In addition to bPI$_3$V, the Respirovirus genus includes the genetically and antigenically related human parainfluenza viruses types 1 and 3 (hPI$_1$V and hPI$_3$V, respectively) and Sendai virus of mice (mPI$_1$V).[6] Like other parainfluenza viruses (PIV), the spherical to pleomorphic 150- to 200-nm bPI$_3$V virion consists of a nucleocapsid surrounded by a lipid envelope that derives from the plasma membrane of the cell from which it buds.[6] bPI$_3$V has a single-stranded, non-segmented, negative-sense RNA genome of 15,456 nucleotides that comprise 6 genes (N-P-M-F-HN-L) that encode for 9 proteins. The conserved N or nucleoprotein, in association with the phosphoprotein (P) and large (L) proteins, together with the genome forms the nucleocapsid or ribonucleoprotein (RNP) core of the virus, which is characteristically helical in form. The P and L proteins, whether associated with the N protein or free in the cytoplasm, are always found in a complex and comprise the viral RNA polymerase that is essential for the transcription of viral mRNA and repli-cation of genomic RNA. The conserved, nonglycosolated matrix, or M protein, is the most abundant viral protein in an infected cell. It is located on the inner face of the envelope and is essential in virus assembly, budding, and release of progeny virions.[7] The homotetrameric hemagglutinin-neuraminidase (HN) and the homotrimeric fusion (F) glycoproteins are in the envelope and mediate attachment to, and penetra-tion of, the host cell, respectively. The domains of these transmembrane proteins that are exposed to the extracellular milieu induce protective antibody responses. The nonstructural, or accessory, V, C, and D proteins result from RNA editing or insertion of G nucleotide residues into the P gene by the viral polymerase. This editing, which results in alternative reading frames, is characteristic of the Paramyxovirinae, and allows 1 gene to encode multiple proteins. The V, C, and D proteins are believed to affect inhibition of interferon α/β in Respirovirus-infected cells.[6]

Studies conducted in the 1960s showed that bPI$_3$V can grow in cells of bovine, porcine, and human origin in vitro, and that this growth was associated with a cyto-pathic effect characterized by plaque formation, syncytia, and eosinophilic intracyto-plasmic inclusion bodies.[8–10] Subsequently, differences in plaque morphology and syncytium formation were reported among bPI$_3$V isolates.[11,12] Differences in neur-aminidase activity, which are somewhat assay dependent, were reported[11–14] among isolates. These differences have been associated with differences in infectivity in vivo; isolates with strong neuraminidase (activity) being able to infect younger calves.[15] Using polyclonal sera in hemagglutination inhibition tests no antigenic differences in the HN protein were reported among bPI$_3$V isolates,[9,10] but, in contrast with initial find-ings,[3] this technique revealed antigenic differences between human and bovine PI$_3$V isolates,[16] the disparity in results apparently being related to the source of sera that were used. Application of monoclonal antibodies in the 1980s and 1990s documented differences among bPI$_3$V isolates,[16,17] primarily in epitopes, in the envelope glycopro-teins HN and F, and significant antigenic differences between human and bovine PI$_3$V isolates.[18,19]

There are few bPI$_3$V genome sequence data.[20–23] Available data[20–23] indicate a high level of genomic conservation among bPI$_3$V isolates tested, the proteins of which, except for the P protein, exhibit 95% or greater identity.[23] There is substantial amino acid sequence identity in N (84%), P (56%), L (84%), M (89%), F (78.5%), and HN (74.6%) proteins between bPI₃V and hPI₃V.[23] A recent study[24] based on partial sequencing of the M protein gene from 7 clinical isolates of bPI₃V and other available sequence data proposed 2 distinct bPI₃V genotypes (bPI₃Va and bPI₃Vb). Aside from the studies on neuraminidase activity and infectivity in small numbers of calves, virtually nothing is known about how reported genetic and antigenic differences may translate into differences in virulence among isolates in cattle.

PATHOGENESIS

Like other respiratory viruses, bPI₃V is spread primarily by large droplet transmission. Once inhaled into the respiratory tract, a bPI₃V virion would first encounter a mucous layer with a high content of N-acetylneuraminic (salic) acid, a natural substrate for the neuraminidase activity of the HN glycoprotein in the viral envelope. Based on early studies conducted with bovine nasal secretions in vitro,[14] it was proposed that the HN molecule in the viral envelope would specifically and sequentially bind to the sialic acid residues in mucus, causing its degradation and effectively allowing the penetration of the virus to subjacent target epithelial cells. This hypothesis has never been formally proven for bPI₃V or other viruses with envelope neuraminidases because of the lack of an appropriate model. Studies with human influenza virus and cultured airway epithelium suggest that neuraminidase activity may remove decoy receptors on mucins, cilia, and the cellular glycocalix, the binding to which could impede viral access to functional receptors on epithelial target cells.[25]

The pathogenesis of bPI₃V infection at the cellular level begins when the HN glycoprotein in the viral envelope, binds to sialic acid residues, probably with specific linkages (α-2,6?) and not indiscriminately,[26] on the glycoproteins and glycolipids of host cells. This is accomplished through the hemagglutination activity of the HN protein that is favored at extracellular (neutral) pH and halide concentration.[6] The ubiquitous presence of the sialic acid receptor molecules explains documented infection of a variety of cell types in the respiratory system. These cells include tracheal cells, ciliated bronchial cells, ciliated and nonciliated bronchiolar cells, and type I and type II pneumoncytes.[27,28] Less well documented, infection of a variety of cells types in the nasal cavity and pharynx is probable. When bound, the HN protein interacts with the F protein, causing a conformational change in the F protein, resulting in fusion between the viral envelope and the host cell membrane.[29] Once fusion occurs, there is a refolding of the proteins in the cell membrane that allows the viral nucleocapsid to enter the cytoplasm.[6] After uncoating or removal of the M protein from the nucleocapsid by an unknown mechanism, viral replication occurs in the cytoplasm and is associated with the presence of intracytoplasmic inclusion bodies[27,28] (**Fig. 1**). This involves, first, viral polymerase-mediated transcription of mRNAs that serve as a template for the translation of viral proteins, and then, after viral proteins accumulate, RNA replication through an intermediate or (plus-stranded) antigenome that is an exact complementary copy of the genome as well as the transcription of mRNAs that serve as a template for the translation of viral proteins.[6] There are 2 notable posttranslational modifications of viral glycoproteins: the first, a prerequisite for viral infectivity, is cleavage of the inactive F protein precursor (F₀) into a fusigenic form comprising F₁ and F₂ subunits that remain linked by disulfide bonds when inserted into plasma membrane. This cleavage is accomplished by endocytotic proteases, notably furin, of the exocytic secretory pathway of the Golgi.[30] The second, which prevents self-binding of viral particles and reattachment to infected cells, and facilitates budding, is the stripping of sialic acid residues from newly formed viral glycoproteins. This process is accomplished

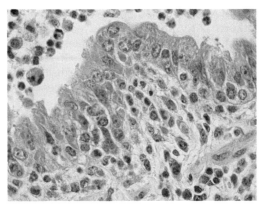

Fig. 1. Eosinophilic intracytoplasmic inclusion bodies characteristic of bPI₃V infection in hyperplastic bronchiolar epithelial cells from a 2-month-old calf 6 days after low-dose aerosol exposure to an in vivo–passaged field isolate of bPI₃V (hematoxylin-eosin stain).

by the neuraminidase activity of HN protein that is favored by the lower pH and halide concentration in intracellular organelles that transport the glycoproteins to the cell surface. The M protein plays multiple roles in the assembly, budding, and release of progeny viruses, including coordinating the assembly and intracellular transport of nucleocapsids to the cell membrane and the transport of F and HN glycoproteins from the endoplasmic reticulum and Golgi to the cell membrane, concentration of viral glycoproteins in the host cell membrane, and bud formation of nascent virions from the host cell plasma membrane.[6] Budding preferentially occurs from the apical (luminal) surface of infected cells.[6,7,27,28]

Although much is now known about the molecular mechanisms of virus-host cell interactions involved in infection and replication of parainfluenza viruses, including bPI₃V, much less is known about the specific nature of cell injury in vivo. Cellular damage may involve different pathways for different parainfluenza viruses in different host species.[6] Recent studies of bPI₃V and hPI₃V infection of bovine and human, respectively,[31,32] in primary cultures of ciliated airway epithelial cells showed little in the way of cytopathology, including syncytium formation.

In contrast, in early, arguably more relevant, studies of bPI₃V-infected tracheal organ cultures from neonatal calves,[33] there was initial reduced epithelial height, loss of cilia, intracytoplasmic inclusion bodies, with swelling and desquamation of superficial cells, followed by epithelial proliferation and syncytium formation. Similar findings were reported in human fetal and adult organ cultures infected with hPI₃V.[34] The epithelial changes in these organ cultures was similar to those reported in the respiratory tract of calves with uncomplicated experimental bPI₃V infections[27,28,35–37] and have been attributed to necrosis.[28] Beyond suggestive morphologic observations, there is no formal proof that bPI₃V-associated cytopathology is caused by necrosis, apoptosis, or programmed cell death, as in the case of Sendai virus (mPI₁V) infection in its natural host, mice,[38] or some other mechanism of cell death,[39] or a combination.

In human medicine, at least in part because of the lack of access to post mortem material from parainfluenza viral–associated illness in children, and equivocal in vitro findings related to virus-induced cytopathology,[32] there has been the suggestion that the immune response plays a role in the pathogenesis of parainfluenza viral infections. This suggestion is supported by the findings of higher concentrations of parainfluenza viral–specific immunoglobulin (Ig) E and histamine release, and increased virus-specific cell-mediated immune responses in infants and children with croup (spasmodic, barking cough) and wheezing compared with cohorts with parainfluenza viral–associated upper respiratory disease,[40] although it is difficult to know whether these are the cause or the effect in severe virus infection. Another area of investigation has been the potential causative role of PIVs in inducing airway hyperresponsiveness. Much of this work has been conducted in laboratory rodents infected with PIVs from other species, which replicate to a limited extent and usually do not cause disease in the xenogeneic host,[6] making interpretation of results difficult. Histamine-associated airway hyperresponsiveness has been reported in a potentially more relevant natural host-virus interaction in canine parainfluenza virus SV5 (genus Rubulavirus)-infected dogs.[41] One study reported increased histamine release from mast cells from the lungs of bPI$_3$V-infected calves.[42] How this may relate to clinical bPI$_3$V-associated respiratory disease, and specifically airway hyperresponsiveness, in cattle is unexamined.

In marked contrast with bovine respiratory syncytial virus (BRSV), the other recognized natural respiratory paramyxoviral infection in cattle, which replicates minimally, if at all, in pulmonary alveolar macrophages (PAM), bPI$_3$V grows to high titer in those important pulmonary immune effector cells.[43] Infection of PAM in vivo was first clearly documented in the classic ultrastructural studies of Bryson and colleagues[28] in the early 1980s. Prior and subsequent studies conducted primarily in vitro with bPI$_3$V-infected PAM showed several functional alterations in the infected cells, including decreased cytotoxicity for virus-infected cells,[44] depression of phagocytosis and bacterial killing,[45,46] and altered arachidonic acid metabolism resulting in secretion of immunosuppressive prostaglandins.[47] An early study reporting decreased proliferative responses by lymphocytes collected from the peripheral blood of bPI$_3$V-infected calves provides some evidence for systemic immunosuppression,[48] although this has not been further examined. bPI$_3$V infection of lymphocytes has been reported in vitro,[49] although no evidence of viral replication was observed in these cells in infected lungs.[28] The multifunctional roles of the accessory proteins C, V, and D in inhibiting the induction of interferon α/β and inhibiting the antiviral intracellular signaling by these interferons has been extensively examined in Sendai virus infection in mice and, to some extent, in hPI$_3$V.[50,51] Suppression of production of β interferon by the V and D proteins of bPI$_3$V has been shown.[52] This antagonism of innate immune responses could also contribute to the pathogenesis of immunosuppression in bPI$_3$V-infected cattle. Taken together with cytopathic effects on the structural components of the mucociliary apparatus, effects of bPI$_3$V on local and systemic immune responses contribute to the establishment of secondary bacterial infections that are a common feature of enzootic pneumonia in calves, and in the bovine respiratory disease (BRD) complex in feedlot cattle.

CLINICAL DISEASE AND LESIONS

A variety of clinical signs of variable severity have been reported in field cases of bPI$_3$V-associated respiratory disease.[1,2,53–56] The common involvement of multiple pathogens in BRD makes it difficult to ascribe signs attributable to bPI$_3$V alone. Attempts to reproduce respiratory disease by intranasal or intratracheal inoculation, or aerosol delivery of bPI$_3$V, or combinations, have yielded mixed results ranging from asymptomatic productive infection to severe pneumonia.[35–37,57,58] Based on a consensus of findings,[5,59] naïve calves develop pyrexia beginning at about 2 days after exposure, which peaks from 40.9 to 41.4°C (104–105°F) on days 4 to 5 and lasts

7 to 10 days. Coughing is often the first presenting clinical sign in field outbreaks[55] and is harsh and hacking. It is coincident with pyrexia.[36] There is also serous to mucopurulent nasal discharge, which indicates rhinitis, and inappetence. Respirations are shallow and rapid (60–70 per minute) and dry expiratory rales may be heard.[36,57] Most uncomplicated bPI$_3$V infections are mild with coughing, nasal discharge, slight fever, and recovery in a few ($\leq$10) days.[59] Clinical disease may be dose dependent in experimental infections.[57] Although it is not possible to definitively diagnose the involvement of bPI$_3$V on clinical findings alone, the presence of a rapid onset of dyspnea is more suggestive of the involvement of BRSV, either alone or in combination with bPI$_3$V.[60]

As with clinical disease, in bPI$_3$V-associated field outbreaks of respiratory disease, evaluation of lesions attributable to bPI$_3$V is usually complicated by the involvement of multiple pathogens, notably *Mannheimia hemolytica* and *Mycoplasma* spp.[53,55,60–63] Experimentally, lesions resulting from bPI$_3$V infection range from rhinitis and tracheitis to severe pneumonia.[35–37,57,58,64] The most severe disease has been reported when young bPI$_3$V-seronegative calves were used as experimental subjects. There may be interisolate differences in pathogenicity or virulence,[35–37,57,58,64] but, aside from a study with 3 isolates differing in neuraminidase activity,[14] this has not been formally evaluated in direct comparative experiments. It has been proposed that there is a dose effect on lesion development,[59] but, as with BRSV,[65] severe pneumonic lesions can be produced with a low dose of in vivo–passaged bPI$_3$V delivered via aerosol (**Fig. 2**), so factors such as degree of attenuation following culture in vitro or route of, or frequency of, challenge[37,58] can affect lesion development.

Grossly, rhinitis may be present, shown by mucopurulent exudate in nasal passage.[58] The gross pneumonic lesions produced by inoculation of bPI$_3$V consist of atelectasis and consolidation in the anterior ventral aspects of lung lobes, especially the more cranial lobes (see **Fig. 2**). These appear initially as swollen and later depressed, red-purple, firm areas that may exude mucopurulent exudate from airways on cut surface.[37,58] There may be interlobular edema.[37,58] Lymph nodes in the chest cavity are usually enlarged and there is no, or minimal, evidence of pleuritis. These gross lung lesions are similar to those produced by experimental infection with BRSV,[65] and are most severe 4 to 16 days after infection.[37] The presence of interlobular emphysema and bullae is a differentiating feature of BRSV infection, and has not been reported in experimental bPI$_3$V infections.

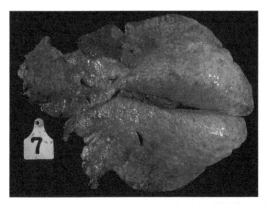

Fig. 2. Acute bronchointerstitial pneumonia in 2-month-old calf 6 days after low-dose aerosol exposure to an in vivo–passaged field isolate of bPI$_3$V. Note red-purple areas of atelectasis and consolidation primarily in the anterior ventral regions of cranial lung lobes.

The histopathologic hallmark of bPI₃V-associated lung lesions is bronchitis/bronchiolitis and alveolitis, characterized by death of a variety of nonciliated and ciliated epithelial cells, beginning as early as 24 hours after infection, with sloughing of effected cells into the lumens of airways[28,37] (**Figs. 1** and **3**). This is accompanied by infiltration by a mixed population of inflammatory cells, which may become severe enough to occlude airways.[37] Intracytoplasmic eosinophilic inclusion bodies are found in bronchial, bronchiolar, and alveolar epithelium (see **Fig. 1**), and are most common between 2 and 7 days after infection.[37] Appearance of epithelial syncytia is more variable, and may be isolate dependent.[35–37] During the repair phase, beginning about 14 days after infection there is hyperplasia of airway and alveolar epithelium.[28,37] There may be organization of bronchiolar exudate leading to bronchiolitis obliterans.[37]

There are only a few reports documenting bPI₃V infection and, rarely, associated disease, outside the respiratory tract of cattle,[35,66–69] prompting the question, What restricts the virus to that body system in most infected animals? It is probably not the phenotype of budding. Although bPI₃V buds primarily from the apical surface of epithelial cells in the respiratory tract,[27,28] the first ultrastructural study of bPI₃V-infected calves[27] documented budding from the basolateral surface, which would allow systemic dissemination of the virus. Once beyond the respiratory tract, there is ubiquity of sialic acid–containing receptor molecules, and cytosolic enzymes that could cleave the F protein precursor (F_0) yield productive systemic infection.[6] Based on evidence of systemic replication of hPI₃V in immunodeficient children,[70,71] it has been proposed[6] that it is the immune response to parainfluenza viruses that restricts infection and disease to the respiratory system in most infected individuals.

BOVINE IMMUNE RESPONSE TO INFECTION

Detection of HI antibodies was a primary observation in the initial discovery of bPI₃V.[1,2] Kinetics of local (predominately IgA) and systemic (predominately IgM and IgG) antibody responses were documented in bPI₃V-seronegative calves that were intranasally inoculated with the virus,[72,73] with both responses being detectable as early as 6 days after infection.[73] VN antibodies in serum were found to persist from 3 to 5 months, whereas antibodies in nasal secretions declined to low or undetectable concentrations by 6 to 8 weeks.[73] Reexposure to bPI₃V resulted in anamnestic serum

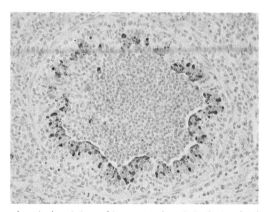

Fig. 3. Immunohistochemical staining of intracytoplasmic inclusion bodies with rabbit anti-bPI₃V serum in epithelial cells in an inflamed bronchiole from a 2-month-old calf 6 days after low-dose aerosol exposure to an in vivo–passaged field isolate of bPI₃V.

and mucosal antibody responses that reached high titer. Nasal antibodies persisted for 5 months, and serum antibodies were detectable for longer.[73] Calves with high concentrations of mucosal antibody and low concentrations of serum antibody were protected from clinical disease following experimental challenge. Those with high serum antibody concentrations and low mucosal antibody were not. Differences in serum or nasal antibody concentrations were also associated with differences in the length of virus nasal shedding.[74] Taken together, it was concluded that mucosal antibody concentrations were more associated with prevention of disease and reduction or prevention of infection, but serum antibody played a role in reducing the severity of disease once it occurred.[73,74] Data concerning antigen specificity of bovine antibody responses to bPI3V are few. One study reported the recognition of proteins with molecular weights consistent with the HN, F, and N proteins by serum antibodies from calves after 1 experimental aerosol exposure to bPI3V.[75] In comparison, natural human infection with hPI3V induces serum antibodies to most viral proteins, but only antibodies reactive with the 2 envelope glycoproteins, HN and F, are virus neutralizing in vitro and in vivo.[76] Antibody responses to HN are usually higher in primary infection, whereas reinfection is often required to stimulate high titers of F-specific serum antibodies.[77] Similar immunologic responses probably are operant in bPI3V-infected cattle.

Given the long-recognized endemicity of bPI3V in cattle populations,[78] most cows usually have serum antibodies that are transferred to calves in colostrum. Early experiments showed that, although colostrum-fed calves became infected, shed virus, and had clinical disease after bPI3V aerosol exposure, the disease was less severe than in colostrum-deprived calves.[79] Nasal antibody resulting from colostral transfer[80] could also contribute to the disease-sparing effect. Calves with maternal antibodies at the time of infection had lower titers of bPI3V-neutralizing antibodies in both serum and nasal secretions 30 days after infection compared with calves that were seronegative at the time of infection,[79] suggesting that passively acquired antibodies suppressed the development of active immunity. Persistence of maternal antibodies was found to be directly associated with initial concentration of transferred antibody.[81] In studies that considered a 1/32 titer of HI antibodies, the threshold of protective immunity, calves with high levels of passive transfer had protective titers until between 19 to 23 weeks of age, whereas the average time of antibody decay to susceptible levels was about 10 weeks.[81]

There continues to be little known about the cell-mediated immune response to bPI3V in cattle,[5] and also to hPI3V in humans.[6] Early work documented delayed hypersensitivity reactions to bPI3V antigens in seropositive cattle that were absent in young calves with passive immunity.[82] Virus-specific lymphocyte proliferative responses and leukocyte migration inhibition have been shown in bPI3V-infected cattle.[83,84] Cells with non–genetically restricted, natural killer cell–like cytotoxic activity against bPI3V-infected cells have been shown in the blood of cattle,[85] as have genetically restricted, cytotoxic lymphocytes (CTL) in the blood of cattle 6 to 9 days after bPI3V infection.[86] Modern tools of investigation of cellular immunity have not been applied to local (pulmonary) responses during bPI3V infection of cattle; however, some extrapolation of results in Sendai virus (mPI1V)–infected mice, and comparison with related infections in cattle, may be instructive. Experimental mPI1V infection of mice, the natural host, results in a rapid increase (5–7 days after infection) in pulmonary CD8+ CTL that coincides with viral clearance and resolution of infection.[87] Similar phenomena have been documented in experimental BRSV infection of cattle.[88] In the mPI1V model, depletion of CD4+ T cells inhibited antibody production, but only marginally delayed viral clearance, again suggesting a critical role for CTL in the recovery from viral infection.[87] In humans, the CD8+ CTL, which are believed to be specific for internal proteins of hPl$_3$V, conferred protection that was weaker and short-lived compared with antibody responses against envelope glycoproteins.[89] In summary, secretory antibodies and CTL probably confer short-lived, incomplete protection against reinfection, whereas virus-neutralizing antibodies in the serum provide long-term disease-sparing effects in the lower respiratory tract.

DIAGNOSTIC APPROACHES

The most definitive ante mortem diagnosis of bPl$_3$V infection is detection of the virus in nasal secretions, best collected on polyester-tipped swabs and transported in medium.[65] Bovine parainfluenza-3 grows readily in bovine turbinate and bovine kidney cells. Identification of the virus in cell culture involves assessment of cytopathic effects, including intracytoplasmic inclusion bodies and syncytium formation, and hemadsorption with guinea pig erythrocytes,[90] or definitive staining using immunofluorescence (IF)[91] or immunohistochemical techniques.[92] As with other paramyxoviruses, such as BRSV, and in contrast with bovine herpes viruses, bPl$_3$V is labile in storage and transport. Failure to appreciate this can result in false-negative isolation results. Rapid diagnosis of bPl$_3$V can also be attempted by IF staining of cells made from smears of nasal swabs.[91]

Acute and convalescent serum samples, optimally 10 to 14 days apart, can be used as an adjunct to antemortem diagnosis of bPl$_3$V infection. Traditionally, this has been accomplished using hemagglutination inhibition or VN tests, but enzyme-linked immunosorbent assays are a more rapid, if less used, alternative.[93] Several factors complicate the use of serology in the diagnosis of bPl$_3$V and other viral respiratory infections of cattle. The endemicity of infection and persistence of maternal antibodies mean that many cattle have antibodies to bPl$_3$V in the absence of recent exposure. Early work documented that some animals with antibody titers (>1/20 HI titer) may not show a serologic response following infection.[74,94] The timing of sampling relative to infection and disease onset can also be an issue.[55,94] Some of these problems could be addressed by the use of an IgM-specific enzyme-linked immunosorbent assay (ELISA) to differentiate recent versus previous exposure to the virus, as has been used with BRSV.[95]

Microscopically or histologically, the presence of bronchiolytic lesions with intracytoplasmic eosinophilic inclusions and, and often syncytia, are suggestive of bPl$_3$V or BRSV infection. These lesions can be differentiated most efficiently and consistently with immunohistochemical staining[92] (**Fig. 3**).

The limitation of any virus detection technique, ante mortem or post mortem, is the timing of sampling after bPl$_3$V infection. In a disease-producing bPl$_3$V experimental infection,[37] the virus could be isolated from the nose for up to 9 days, and the lung for up to 12 days, after infection, under optimal handling and transport conditions that are unlikely to be practiced in many field situations; staining methods are likely to be less sensitive. By the time that many, if not most, calves die of enzootic pneumonia or BRD in the feedlot, often after 1 or more treatment attempts, bPl$_3$V would be gone. This timing probably results in false-negative results or underestimates of the involvement of bPl$_3$V when specific causal diagnoses are attempted on material collected at post mortem.[62,63] Notwithstanding the limitations of serology, stored paired serum samples may be the only way to document the involvement of bPl$_3$V in outbreak situations when virus detection attempts are not undertaken or fail to yield positive results.[96]

EPIDEMIOLOGY

From the time of its discovery to the present, bPl$_3$V has been recognized to be endemic in beef and dairy cattle populations whenever and wherever investigated.[1,2,54,55,59,78,97–99]

Most of the epidemiologic investigations have been conducted in housed calves in Europe. Aside from a recent study in Mexico[98] and a few prevalence (of bPI$_3$V antibody) studies in feedlot cattle, there have been no published epidemiologic investigations of bPI$_3$V in North America for more than 30 years. This makes it difficult to know how changes in cattle production, including the intensification of the dairy and feedlot industries, may have affected the epidemiology of bPI$_3$V infection. Historically, antibody titers to bPI$_3$V increase in prevalence and magnitude with increasing age of animals.[59,78] Most reports of natural and experimental disease have been in young animals, which could be reflective of immune status. Subclinical infections have been reported[59,78] and are most likely underappreciated, but contribute to both transmission and the maintenance of herd immunity. The duration of immunity to bPI$_3$V infection is not known. Experimentally, seropositive calves can be reinfected several weeks after primary exposure.[57] They may or may not excrete virus, but, if virus excretion does occur, it is usually of shorter duration than in primary infection.[57] In naturally occurring bPI$_3$V infection, virus could be isolated from individual calves for a period of months. It was not determined whether this indicated a persistent primary infection or reinfection.[55,97]

In temperate climates, infection and disease occur most commonly in autumn and winter months,[78,97] and often occur with other acute respiratory virus infections.[54,62,68,78,96,97] Infection probably most commonly occurs via the respiratory route, being transmitted in nasal mucous, ocular secretions, and droplets, and is therefore enhanced by crowding in calf barns, auction markets, and during transport.[59,78] The infectious dose of bPI$_3$V is not known, but is likely to be much lower than the concentration of virus in nasal secretions, which can be as high as 10^6 to $10^{7.5}$ TCID$_{50}$ (the median tissue culture infective dose)/mL, peaking about 4 days after experimental infection.[59] By comparison, two-thirds of adult, moderately seropositive human volunteers became infected and developed coldlike symptoms following the intranasal instillation of only 80 TCID$_{50}$ of hPI$_1$V.[100] Experimentally, bPI$_3$V is stable and infectious in droplets of nasal secretions for at least 3 hours, and viability is enhanced by cold temperatures (6°C).[101] The true duration of infectivity of bPI$_3$V in environmental conditions is not known.

One of the most intriguing and unresolved issues in the biology of paramyxovirus infections is the potential for cross-species infection. Antibodies reactive with bPI$_3$V have been reported in several, mostly ungulate, species.[24,78] Biologic assays such as HI and VN using polyclonal antibodies are likely to detect cross-reactive responses.[102] Cross-reactive responses are more likely if an animal has been repeatedly exposed to the same PIV, or a different, related PIV.[102] Induction of cross-reactive antibodies to PIVs can confound seroepidemiology. Without sequencing of viral isolates, it is not possible to determine whether bPI$_3$V-reactive antibodies are the result of infection with bPI$_3$V or infection with a species-divergent PIV that is related to bPI$_3$V. Nevertheless, it has long been recognized that bPI$_3$V, or bPI$_3$V-like viruses, can infect and cause disease in sheep, including wild sheep.[66,103–105] Conversely, ovine bPI$_3$V-like isolates can cause disease in calves.[104] The prevalence and importance of bPI$_3$V-like viruses in goats is less well documented.[106] There are scant data indicating genetic differences among bovine and ovine bPI$_3$V-like isolates.[107] It is likely that both are members of the same cross-infecting quasispecies, which may also include other ungulate viruses.[6] Recently bPI$_3$V-like viruses were isolated from pigs with neurologic signs.[108] Although they produced mild respiratory disease following intranasal infection of pigs in prospective transmission experiments, it was concluded, based on negative results in a serosurvey of pigs in Minnesota and Iowa, that they were variants of bPI$_3$V that infected pigs but failed to establish an enzootic state.[108]

From a public health perspective, there is 1 report of respiratory disease in a human adolescent putatively caused by bPI$_3$V.[109] This association was made because higher HI and complement-fixing antibodies to bPI$_3$V compared with hPI$_3$V in that patient, and not on isolation and identification of the causative virus. Although the potential for human infection by bPI$_3$V has been acknowledged, it has been, and still is, generally believed that bPI$_3$V is not a serious zoonotic concern.[6,78] bPI$_3$V replicates and causes mild respiratory disease in humans and nonhuman primates.[110] It has been used successfully in a so-called Jennerian approach (ie, using a closely related agent from 1 species to protect from disease caused by the cognate pathogen in the vaccinee) to protect against hPI$_3$V-associated disease in primates, including humans, and is therefore considered as a vaccine candidate for hPI$_3$V.[6,110,111] There are scant and conflicting data regarding the ability of hPI$_3$V to infect and cause disease in cattle.[78]

CONTROL AND PROPHYLAXIS

As with other respiratory pathogens, early observations on naturally occurring outbreaks suggested or documented the role of environmental factors, notably poor ventilation in housed calves, or the stresses of the feedlot environment, in maximizing the severity of respiratory disease problems associated with bPI$_3$V.[1,2,59,78] Attention to good husbandry practices are essential in controlling the transmission of bPI$_3$V, and the severity of disease once transmission has occurred.

Development of vaccines for bPI$_3$V began in the 1960s, soon after its discovery.[112] Parenteral inactivated vaccines developed in the 1960s and 1970s, at least 1 of which used an hPI$_3$V,[112] were generally shown to stimulate systemic, and sometimes local, antibody responses after 2 doses to calves with no or low antibodies.[112–114] The antibody response was associated with reduced viral shedding after challenge. The development and testing of modified live virus (MLV) vaccines for bPI$_3$V, both parenteral, first, and then intranasal delivery, also began in the 1960s and continues to the present.[58,74,112,115–120] Current bPI$_3$V-containing vaccines are generally combination vaccines containing 1 or more other viruses, and sometimes bacteria. Current intranasal bPI$_3$V vaccines routinely use temperature-sensitive mutants that would have restricted, if any, replication in the lower respiratory tract.[118,120] Although both types of vaccines have generally been shown to stimulate both local and systemic antibody responses, this is dependent on the status of local and systemic antibody concentrations at the time of vaccination.[58,74,112,115–120] There are conflicting data deriving from early direct comparisons of the relative efficacy of parenteral versus intranasal MLV vaccines. Some[74,115] reported better protection against experimental infection following intranasal vaccination, and another[116] found no advantage of one compared with the other. Available recent data indicate the inhibitory effect of maternal antibodies on the development of active immunity to parenterally delivered combination MLV vaccines containing bPI$_3$V.[121,122] The most recent study indicates that systemic VN titers to bPI$_3$V must decline to between 1:8 and 1:16 before 90% of calves will respond positively to parenteral vaccination by day 28 after vaccination. For a response by 14 days after vaccination, a lower titer of 1:4 at the time of vaccination is required.[122] Some studies have suggested[116] or shown[120] that the intranasal route is more likely to overcome the inhibiting effect of maternal antibodies in young calves. Aside from some evidence that intranasal bPI$_3$V vaccine can enhance chemotactic activity of PAM following challenge,[123] little known about the cell-mediated immune response to bPI$_3$V vaccines. In addition, little is known about the optimal protocol for primary immunization and boosting, or the duration of immunity (DOI) of the various bPI$_3$V vaccines. In one recent study of a European combination parenteral MLV vaccine, the DOI of the bPI$_3$V component was at least 6 months, as determined by an increase in VN antibody titer and reduction in bPI$_3$V shedding in vaccinated versus control calves that were 6 to 7 months old at the time of initial vaccination in a 2-dose protocol.[124]

A problem in comparatively evaluating laboratory studies of the efficacy of the bPI$_3$V component of various vaccines is inconsistency in bPI$_3$V challenge models. With regard to reproduction of disease; there often has not been any. This problem is compounded in North America where the criteria for a satisfactory test in the current US Department of Agriculture guidelines for the licensure of bPI$_3$V vaccines only require an increase in systemic VN antibody titer to 1:4 after vaccination, and a significant reduction in nasal shedding of the virus compared with unvaccinated controls. Production and evaluation of disease is not a requirement.[125] It has been more than 30 years since there has been any published challenge study concerning bPI$_3$V vaccines used in North America. Evaluation of the bPI$_3$V component of vaccines in field trials is also difficult, even if they are well-designed trials,[126–128] primarily because enzootic pneumonia and BRD are multifactorial, and documentation of the involvement of bPI$_3$V can be difficult, if it is attempted at all. Notwithstanding all of these concerns and deficits in knowledge, priming mucosally early in calfhood with intranasal vaccine, followed by boosting parenterally when maternal antibodies have decayed at 2 to 3 months of age, may be the best approach to immunoprophylaxis.

SUMMARY

bPI$_3$V is a long-recognized, currently underappreciated, endemic infection in dairy and beef cattle populations. Clinical disease is most common in calves with poor passive transfer or decayed maternal antibodies. It is usually mild, consisting of fever, nasal discharge, and dry cough. Caused at least partly by local immunosuppressive effects, bPI$_3$V infection is often complicated by coinfection with other respiratory viruses and bacteria, and is therefore an important component of enzootic pneumonia in calves and BRD in feedlot cattle. Active infection can be diagnosed by virus isolation from nasal swabs, or IF testing on smears made from nasal swabs. Acute and convalescent serum samples and HI, VN, or tests can be used as adjunct diagnostic approaches. Microscopically typical bronchiolytic lesions containing intracytoplasmic inclusion bodies and syncytia can be differentiated from BRSV infection using immunohistochemistry. Timing of sampling is critical in obtaining definitive diagnostic test results. Parenteral and intranasal MLV combination vaccines are available. Although not formally examined, priming early in calfhood with intranasal vaccine, followed by boosting with parenteral vaccine, may be the best immunoprophylactic approach.

REFERENCES

1. Reisinger RC, Heddleston KL, Manthei CA. A myxovirus (SF-4) associated with shipping fever of cattle. J Am Vet Med Assoc 1959;135:147–52.
2. Hoerlein AB, Mansfield ME, Abinati FR, et al. Studies of shipping fever of cattle. I. Para-influenza 3 virus antibodies in feeder calves. J Am Vet Med Assoc 1959; 135:153–60.
3. Abinanti FR, Huebner RJ. The serological relationships of strains of parainfluenza 3 virus isolated from humans and cattle with respiratory disease. Virology 1959;8:391–4.

4. Andrewes CH, Bang FB, Chanock RM, et al. Para-influenza viruses 1, 2, and 3: suggested names for recently described myxoviruses. Virology 1959;8:129–30, 6c.
5. Kapil S, Basaraba RJ. Infectious bovine rhinotracheitis, parainfluenza-3, and respiratory coronavirus. Vet Clin North Am Food Anim Pract 1997;13:455–69.
6. Karron RA, Collins PL. Parainfluenza viruses. In: Knipe DM, Howley PM, editors. 5th edition, Fields virology, vol. 1. Philadelphia: Lippincott, Williams & Wilkins; 2007. p. 1497–526.
7. Takimoto T, Portner A. Molecular mechanism of paramyxovirus budding. Virus Res 2004;106:133–45.
8. Dinter Z, Hermondsson S, Bakos K. Studies on variants of a bovine strain of parainfluenza-3 virus (1) isolation and growth characteristics. Acta Pathol Microbiol Scand 1960;49:485–92.
9. McKercher MG. A comparative study of a strain of myxovirus from cattle in California affected with shipping fever with American and European strains of parainfluenza 3 virus. Cornell Vet 1963;53:262–9.
10. Burroughs AI, Suleiman PP. Forty-one isolates of parainfluenza-3 virus from dairy and beef cattle compared. Cornell Vet 1963;53:262–9.
11. Shibuta H, Kanda T, Hazama A, et al. Parainfluenza 3 virus: plaque-type variants lacking neuraminidase activity. Infect Immun 1981;34:262–7.
12. Shibuta H, Nozawa A, Shioda T, et al. Neuraminidase activity and syncytial formation in variants of parainfluenza 3 virus. Infect Immun 1983;41:780–8.
13. Drzeniek R, Bogel K, Roll R. On the classification of bovine parainfluenza-3 viruses. Virology 1967;31:725–7.
14. Morein B, Bergman R. Effect of parainfluenza-3 neuraminidase on bovine nasal secretion. Infect Immun 1972;6:174–7.
15. Bergman R, Moreno-Lopez J, Mollerberg L, et al. Parainfluenza-3 virus: difference in capacity of neuraminidase weak and strong strains to infect young calves and to elicit cellular immune response. Res Vet Sci 1978;25:193–9.
16. Ketler A, Hamparian VV, Hilleman MR. Laboratory and field investigations of bovine myxovirus parainfluenza 3 virus and vaccine. I. Properties of the SF-4 (shipping fever) strain of virus. J Immunol 1961;87:126–33.
17. Shibuta H, Suzu S, Shioda T. Differences in bovine parainfluenza 3 virus variants studied by monoclonal antibodies against viral glycoproteins. Virology 1986; 155:688–96.
18. Ray R, Compans RW. Monoclonal antibodies reveal extensive antigenic differences between the hemaglutinin-neuraminidase glycoproteins of human and bovine parainfluenza 3 viruses. Virology 1986;148:232–6.
19. Klippmark E, Rydbeck R, Shibuta H, et al. Antigenic variation of human and bovine parainfluenza virus type 3 strains. J Gen Virol 1990;71:1577–80.
20. Sakai Y, Suzu S, Shioda T, et al. Nucleotide sequence of the bovine parainfluenza 3 genome: its 3′end and the genes of NP, P, C and M proteins. Nucleic Acids Res 1987;15:2927–44.
21. Shioda T, Wakao S, Suzu S, et al. Differences in bovine parainfluenza 3 virus variants studied by sequencing of the genes of viral envelope proteins. Virology 1988;162:388–96.
22. Breker-Klassen MM, Yoo D, Babiuk LA. Comparisons of the F and HN gene sequences of different strains of bovine parainfluenza virus type 3: relationship to phenotype and pathogenicity. Can J Vet Res 1996;60:228–36.
23. Bailly JE, McAuliffe JM, Skiadopoulos MH, et al. Sequence determination and molecular analysis of two strains of bovine parainfluenza virus type 3 that are attenuated for primates. Virus Genes 2000;20:173–82.

24. Harwood PF, Gravel LJ, Mahony TJ. Identification of two distinct bovine parainfluenza virus type 3 genotypes. J Gen Virol 2008;89:1643–8.

25. Matrosovich MN, Matrosovich TY, Gray T, et al. Neuraminidase is important for the initiation of influenza virus infection in human airway epithelium. J Virol 2004;78:12665–7.

26. Levin Perlman S, Jordan M, Brossmer R, et al. The use of a quantitative fusion assay to evaluate HN-receptor interaction for human parainfluenza virus type 3. Virology 1999;265:57–65.

27. Tsai KS, Thomson RG. Bovine parainfluenza type 3 virus infection: Ultrastructural aspects of viral pathogenesis in the bovine respiratory tract. Infect Immun 1975;11:783–803.

28. Bryson DG, McNulty MS, McCracken RM, et al. Ultrastructural features of experimental parainfluenza type 3 virus pneumonia in calves. J Comp Pathol 1983;93:397–414.

29. Lamb RA, Paterson RG, Jardetzky TS. Paramyxovirus membrane fusion: lessons from the F and HN atomic structures. Virology 2006;344:30–7.

30. Nagai Y. Virus activation by host proteinases. A pivotal role in the spread of infection, tissue tropism and pathogenicity. Microbiol Immunol 1995;39:1–9.

31. Goris K, Uhlenbeck S, Schwegmann-Wessels C, et al. Differential sensitivity of differentiated epithelial cells to respiratory viruses reveals different viral strategies of host infection. J Virol 2009;83:1962–8.

32. Zhang L, Bukreyev A, Thompson CI, et al. Infection of ciliated cells by human parainfluenza virus type 3 in an in vitro model of human airway epithelium. J Virol 2005;79:1113–24.

33. Campbell RS, Thompson H, Leighton E, et al. Pathogenesis of bovine parainfluenza 3 virus infection in organ cultures. J Comp Pathol 1969;79:347–54.

34. Craighead JE, Brennan BJ. Cytopathic effects of parainfluenza virus type 3 in organ cultures of human respiratory tract tissue. Am J Pathol 1968;52:287–300.

35. Dawson PS, Derbyshire JH, Lamont PH. The inoculation of calves with parainfluenza-3 virus. Res Vet Sci 1965;6:108–13.

36. Omar AR, Jennings AR, Betts AO. The experimental disease produced in calves by the J121 strain of parainfluenza virus type 3. Res Vet Sci 1966;7:379–88.

37. Bryson DG, McNulty MS, Ball HJ, et al. The experimental production of pneumonia in calves by intranasal inoculation of parainfluenza type-3 virus. Vet Rec 1979;105:566–73.

38. Garcin D, Taylor G, Tanebayashi K, et al. The short Sendai virus leader region controls induction of programmed cell death. Virology 1998;243:340–53.

39. Fink SL, Cookson BT. Apoptosis, pyroptosis, and necrosis: mechanistic description of dead and dying eukaryotic cells. Infect Immun 2005;73:1907–16.

40. Welliver RC, Wong DT, Middleton E Jr, et al. Role of parainfluenza virus-specific IgE in the pathogenesis of croup and wheezing subsequent to infection. J Pediatr 1982;101:889–96.

41. Lemen RJ, Quan SF, Witten ML, et al. Canine parainfluenza type 2 bronchiolitis increases histamine responsiveness in beagle puppies. Am Rev Respir Dis 1990;141:199–207.

42. Ogunbiyi PO, Black WD, Eyre P. Parainfluenza-3 virus-induced enhancement of histamine release from calf lung mast cells–effect of levamisole. J Vet Pharmacol Ther 1988;11:338–44.

43. Schrijver RS, Kramps JA, Middel WG, et al. Bovine respiratory syncytial virus replicates minimally in bovine alveolar macrophages. Arch Virol 1995;140:1905–17.

44. Probert M, Stott EJ, Thomas LH. Interactions between calf alveolar macrophages and parainfluenza-3 virus. Infect Immun 1976;15:576–85.
45. Liggitt D, Huston L, Silflow R, et al. Impaired function of bovine alveolar macrophages infected with parainfluenza-3 virus. Am J Vet Res 1985;46:1740–4.
46. Slauson DO, Ley JC, Castleman WL, et al. Alveolar macrophage phagocytic kinetics following pulmonary parainfluenza-3 virus infection. J Leukoc Biol 1987;41:412–20.
47. Laegreid WW, Taylor SM, Leid RW, et al. Virus-induced enhancement of arachidonate metabolism by bovine alveolar macrophages in vitro. J Leukoc Biol 1989;45:283–92.
48. Pospisil Z, Machatkova M, Mensik J, et al. Decline in the phytohaemagglutinin responsiveness of lymphocytes from calves infected experimentally with bovine viral diarrhoea-mucosal disease virus and parainfluenza 3 virus. Acta Vet Brno 1975;44:369–75.
49. Basaraba RJ, Laegreid WW, Brown PR, et al. Cell-to-cell contact not soluble factors mediate suppression of lymphocyte proliferation by bovine parainfluenza virus type 3. Viral Immunol 1994;7:121–32.
50. Komatsu T, Takeuchi K, Yokoo A, et al. C and V proteins of Sendai virus target signalling pathways leading to IRF-3 activation for the negative regulation of interferon-beta production. Virology 2004;325:137–48.
51. Durbin AP, McAuliffe JM, Collins PL, et al. Mutations in the C, D, and V open reading frames of human parainfluenza virus type 3 attenuate replication in rodents and primates. Virology 1999;261:319–30.
52. Komatsu T, Takeuchi K, Gotoh B. Bovine parainfluenza virus type 3 accessory proteins that suppress beta interferon production. Microbes Infect 2007;9:954–62.
53. Betts AO, Jennings AR, Omar AR, et al. Pneumonia in calves caused by parainfluenza virus type 3. Vet Rec 1964;76:382–4.
54. Rosenquist BD, Dobson AW. Multiple viral infection in calves with acute bovine respiratory tract disease. Am J Vet Res 1974;34:363–5.
55. Allen EM, Pirie HM, Selman IE, et al. Some characteristics of a natural infection by parainfluenza-3 virus in a group of calves. Res Vet Sci 1978;24:339–46.
56. Bryson EG, McFerran JB, Ball HJ, et al. Observations on outbreaks of respiratory disease in housed calves. 1. Epidemiological, clinical and microbiological findings. Vet Rec 1978;103:485–9.
57. Frank GH, Marshall RG. Relationship of serum and nasal secretion neutralizing antibodies in protection of calves against parainfluenza-3 virus. Am J Vet Res 1971;32:1707–13.
58. Bryson DG, Adair BM, McNulty MS, et al. Studies on the efficacy of intranasal vaccination for the prevention of experimentally induced parainfluenza type 3 virus pneumonia in calves. Vet Rec 1999;145:33–9.
59. Frank GH, Marshall RG. Parainfluenza-3 virus infection of cattle. J Am Vet Med Assoc 1973;163:858–60.
60. Bryson EG, McFerran JB, Ball HJ, et al. Observations on outbreaks of respiratory disease in calves associated with parainfluenza type 3 virus and respiratory syncytial virus infection. Vet Rec 1979;104:45–9.
61. Bryson EG, McFerran JB, Ball HJ, et al. Observations on outbreaks of respiratory disease in housed calves. 2. Pathological and microbiological findings. Vet Rec 1978;103:5503–9.
62. Fulton RW, Purdy CW, Confer AW, et al. Bovine viral diarrhea infections in feeder calves with respiratory disease: interactions with *Pasteruella* spp., parainfluenza-3 virus, and bovine respiratory syncytial virus. Can J Vet Res 2000;64:151–9.

63. Gagea M, Bateman KG, van Drumel T, et al. Diseases and pathogens associated with mortality in Ontario beef feedlots. J Vet Diagn Invest 2006;18:18–28.

64. Bögel K. [Virological findings in calves with respiratory syndrome with special reference to parainfluenza virus type 3]. Monatshefte für Tierheilkunde 1961; 13:129–35 [in German].

65. West K, Petrie L, Haines DM, et al. The effect of formalin-inactivated vaccine on respiratory disease associated with bovine respiratory syncytial virus infection in calves. Vaccine 1999;17:809–20.

66. Woods GT, Sibinovic K, Marquis G. Experimental exposure of calves, lambs, and colostrum-deprived pigs to bovine myxovirus parainfluenza-3. Am J Vet Res 1965;26:52–6.

67. Hamdy AH. Association of myxovirus PI3 with pneumoenteritis of calves-virus isolation. Am J Vet Res 1966;27:981–6.

68. Van der Maaten. Immunofluorescent studies of bovine parainfluenza-3 virus in experimentally infected calves. Can J Comp Med 1969;33:141–7.

69. Swift BL, Kennedy PC. Experimentally induced infection of in utero bovine fetuses with bovine parainfluenza 3 virus. Am J Vet Res 1972;33:57–63.

70. Fishaut M, Tubergen D, McIntosh K. Cellular response to respiratory viruses with particular reference to children with disorders of cell-mediated immunity. J Pediatr 1980;96:179–86.

71. Frank JA Jr, Warren RW, Tucker JA, et al. Disseminated parainfluenza infection in a child with severe combined immunodeficiency. Am J Dis Child 1983;137: 1172–4.

72. Morein B. Immunity against parainfluenza-3 virus in cattle; immunglobulins in serum and nasal secretions. Int Arch Allergy 1970;39:403–14.

73. Marshall RG, Frank GH. Neutralising antibody in serum and nasal secretions of calves exposed to parainfluenza-3 virus. Am J Vet Res 1971;32:1669–706.

74. Gates GA, Cesario TC, Ebert JW, et al. Neutralising antibody in experimentally induced respiratory virus infection in calves. Am J Vet Res 1970;31:217–24.

75. Toth TE, Frank GH. Bovine parainfluenza-3 virus proteins recognized by antibodies of aerosol-exposed calves. Am J Vet Res 1988;49:1945–9.

76. Kasel JA, Frank AL, Keitel WA, et al. Acquisition of serum antibodies to specific viral glycoproteins of parainfluenza-3 in children. J Virol 1964;52:828–32.

77. van Wyke Coelingh KL, Winter CC, Tierney EL, et al. Antibody responses of humans and nonhuman primates to individual antigenic sites of the hemagglutinin-neuraminidase and fusion glycoproteins after primary infection or reinfection with parainfluenza type 3 virus. J Virol 1990;64:3833–43.

78. Woods GT. The natural history of bovine myxovirus parainfluenza-3. J Am Vet Med Assoc 1968;152:771–6.

79. Marshall RG, Frank GH. Clinical and immunological responses of calves with colostrally acquired maternal antibody against parainfluenza-3 virus to homologous viral challenge. Am J Vet Res 1975;36:1085–9.

80. McKercher DG. Nasal versus parenteral vaccination for the protection of cattle against viral infection of the respiratory tract. Arch Vet Ital 1972;23:63–74.

81. Dawson PS. Persistence of maternal antibodies to parainfluenza 3 virus. J Comp Path 1966;76:373–8.

82. Morein B, Moren-Lopez JW. Skin hypersensitivity to parainfluenza-3 virus (PIV3) in cattle. Zentralbl Veterinaermed 1973;20:540–6.

83. Moren-Lopez JW. Cell-mediated immunity to parainfluenza-3 virus (PIV3) in cattle. Evaluation of in vivo and in vitro tests. Zentralbl Veterinaermed B 1977; 24:231–40.

84. Johnson K, Morein B. *In vitro* stimulation of bovine circulating lymphocytes by parainfluenza type 3 virus. Res Vet Sci 1977;22:83–5.

85. Campos M, Rossi CR, Lawman MJ. Natural cell-mediated cytotoxicity of bovine mononuclear cells against virus-infected cells. Infect Immun 1982;36:1054–9.

86. Bamford AI, Adair BM, Foster JC. Primary cytotoxic response of bovine peripheral blood leukocytes to parainfluenza type 3 virus infection. Vet Immunol Immunopathol 1995;45:85–95.

87. Hou S, Doherty PC, Zijlstra M, et al. Delayed clearance of Sendai virus in mice lacking class I MHC-restricted CD8+ T cells. J Immunol 1992;129:1319–25.

88. West K, Petrie L, Konoby C, et al. The efficacy of modified-live bovine respiratory syncytial virus vaccines in experimentally infected calves. Vaccine 1999;18:907–19.

89. Tao T, Davoodi F, Cho CJ, et al. A live attenuated recombinant chimeric parainfluenza virus (PIV) candidate vaccine containing the hemagglutinin-neuraminidase and fusion glycoproteins of PIV1 and the remaining proteins from PIV3 induces resistance to PIV1 even in animals immune to PIV3. Vaccine 2000;18:1359–66.

90. Minnich LL, Ray CG. Early testing of cell cultures for detection of hemadsorbing viruses. J Clin Microbiol 1987;25:421–2.

91. McFerran JB, McNulty MS. Aids to diagnosis of virological diseases. Br Vet J 1981;137:455–63.

92. Haines DM, Kendall JC, Remenda BW, et al. Monoclonal and polyclonal antibodies for immunohistochemical detection of bovine parainfluenza type 3 virus in frozen and formalin-fixed paraffin-embedded tissues. J Vet Diagn Invest 1992;4:393–9.

93. Graham DA, McShane J, Mawhinney KA, et al. Evaluation of a single dilution ELISA system for detection of seroconversion to bovine viral diarrhea, bovine respiratory syncytial virus, parainfluenza-3 virus, and infectious rhinotracheitis virus: comparison with testing by virus neutralization and hemagglutination inhibition. J Vet Diagn Invest 1998;10:43–8.

94. Thomas LH. Observations on the role of viruses in pneumonia of calves. Vet Rec 1973;93:384–8.

95. Westenbrink F, Kimman TG. Immunoglobulin M specific enzyme-linked immunosorbent assay for serodiagnosis of bovine respiratory syncytial virus infections. Am J Vet Res 1987;48:1132–7.

96. Allen JW, Viel L, Bateman KG, et al. Serological titers to bovine herpesvirus 1, bovine viral diarrhea virus, parainfluenza 3 virus, bovine respiratory syncytial virus and *Pasteurella haomolytioa* in foodlot calves with respiratory disease: associations with bacteriological and pulmonary cytological variables. Can J Vet Res 1992;56:281–8.

97. Stott EJ, Thomas LH, Collins AP, et al. A survey of virus infections of the respiratory tract of cattle and their association with disease. J Hyg (Camb) 1980;85:257–70.

98. Solis-Calderon JJ, Segura-Correa JC, Aguilar-Romero F, et al. Detection of antibodies and risk factors for infection with bovine respiratory syncytial virus and parainfluenza virus-3 in beef cattle of Yucatan, Mexico. Prev Vet Med 2007;82:102–10.

99. Gulliksen SM, Jor E, Lie KI, et al. Respiratory infections in Norwegian dairy calves. J Dairy Sci 2009;92:5139–46.

100. Smith CB, Purcell RH, Bellanti JA, et al. Protective effect of antibody to parainfluenza type 1 virus. N Engl J Med 1966;275:1145–52.

101. Elazhary MA, Derbyshire JB. Aersosol stability of bovine parainfluenza type 3 virus. Can J Comp Med 1979;43:295–304.

102. Cook KM, Andrews BE, Fox HH, et al. Antigenic relationships among the "newer" myxoviruses (parainfluenza). Am J Hyg 1959;69:250–64.

103. Hore DE. Isolation of ovine strains of parainfluenza virus serologically related to type 3. Vet Rec 1966;79:466–7.

104. Stevenson RG, Hore DE. Comparative pathology of lambs and calves infected with parainfluenza virus type 3. J Comp Path 1970;80:613–8.

105. Rudolph KM, Hunter DL, Rimler RB, et al. Microorganisms associated with a pneumonic epizootic in Rocky Mountain bighorn sheep (Ovis canadensis canadensis). J Zoo Wildl Med 2007;38:548–58.

106. Yener Z, Saglam YS, Timurkaan N, et al. Immunohistochemical detection of parainfluenza type 3 virus antigens in paraffin sections of pneumonic caprine lungs. J Vet Med A Physiol Pathol Clin Med 2005;52:268–71.

107. Lyon M, Leroux C, Greenland T, et al. Presence of a unique parainfluenza virus 3 strain identified by RT-PCR in visna-maedi virus infected sheep. Vet Microbiol 1997;57:95–104.

108. Qia D, Janke BH, Elankumaran S. Complete genomic sequence and pathogenicity of two swine parainfluenza 3 isolates from pigs in the United States. J Virol 2010;84:686–94.

109. Ben-Ishai Z, Naftali V, Avram A, et al. Human infection by a bovine strain of parainfluenza virus type 3. J Med Virol 1980;6:165–8.

110. Schmidt AC, McAuliffe JM, Huang A, et al. Bovine parainfluenza virus type 3 (BPIV3) fusion and hemagglutinin-neuraminidase glycoproteins make an important contribution to the restricted replication of BPIV3 in primates. J Virol 2000;74:8922–9.

111. Sato M, Wright PF. Current status of vaccines for parainfluenza virus infections. Pediatr Infect Dis J 2008;27:S123–5.

112. Gale C. Bovine parainfluenza-3 immunization procedures. J Am Vet Med Assoc 1968;152:871–80.

113. Morein B. Immunity against parainfluenza-3 virus in cattle; immunoglobulins in serum and nasal secretions after subcutaneous and nasal vaccination. Z Immunitatsforch Exp Klin Immunol 1972;144:63–74.

114. Probert M, Stott EJ, Thomas LH, et al. An inactivated parainfluenza virus type 3 vaccine; the influence of vaccination regime on the response of calves and their subsequent resistance to challenge. Res Vet Sci 1978;24:222–7.

115. Gutekunst D, Paton I, Volenec F. Parainfluenza-3 vaccine in cattle: comparative efficacy of intranasal and intramuscular routes. J Am Vet Med Assoc 1969;155:1879–85.

116. McKercher DG, Saito JK, Franti, et al. Response of calves to parainfluenza-3 vaccines administered nasally or parenterally. J Am Vet Med Assoc 1972;33:721–30.

117. Woods GT, Crandall RA, Mansfield ME. A comparison of immunologic response to intranasal and intramuscular parainfluenza-3 live virus vaccines in beef calves challenged experimentally in the feedlot. Res Commun Chem Pathol Pharmacol 1975;11:117–28.

118. Zygraich N, Labmann M, Peetermens J, et al. In vivo and in vitro characteristics of a ts mutant of bovine parainfluenza 3 virus in "Imuresp P" vaccine. Tieraerztl Umsch 1979;34:555–62.

119. Salt JS, Thevasagayam SJ, Wiseman A, et al. Efficacy of a quadrivalent vaccine against respiratory diseases caused by BHV-1, PI3V, BVDV and BRSV in experimentally infected calves. Vet J 2007;174:616–26.

120. Vangeel I, Ioannou F, Riegler L, et al. Efficacy of an intranasal modified live bovine respiratory syncytial virus and temperature-sensitive parainfluenza type 3 virus vaccine in 3-week-old calves experimentally challenged with PI3V. Vet J 2009;179:101–8.
121. Adair BM, Bradford HE, Bryson DG, et al. Effect of parainfluenza-3 virus challenge on cell-mediated immune function in parainfluenza-3 vaccinated and non-vaccinated calves. Res Vet Sci 2000;68:197–9.
122. Fulton RW, Briggs RE, Payton ME, et al. Maternally derived humoral immunity to bovine viral diarrhea virus (BVDV) 1a, BVDV1b, BVDV2, bovine herpesvirus-1, parainfluenza-3 virus bovine respiratory syncytial virus, *Mannheimia haemolytica* and *Pasteurella multocida* in beef calves, antibody decline by half-life studies and effect on response to vaccination. Vaccine 2004;22:643–9.
123. O'Neill RG, Fitzpatrick JL, Glass EJ, et al. Optimisation of the response to respiratory virus vaccines in cattle. Vet Rec 2007;161:269–70.
124. Peters AR, Thevasagayam SJ, Wiseman A, et al. Duration of immunity of a quadrivalent vaccine against respiratory diseases caused by BHV-1, PI3V, BVDV, and BRSV in experimentally infected calves. Prev Vet Med 2004;66:63–77.
125. Bovine parainfluenza3 vaccine. 9CFR 113.309.
126. Martin SW. Vaccination: is it effective in preventing respiratory disease or influencing weight gains in feedlot cattle. Can Vet J 1983;24:10–9.
127. Schunicht OC, Booker CW, Jim GK, et al. Comparison of a multivalent viral vaccine program versus a univalent viral vaccine program on animal health, feedlot performance, and carcass characteristics of feedlot calves. Can Vet J 2003;44:43–50.
128. Stilwell G, Matos M, Carolino N, et al. Effect of a quadrivalent vaccine against respiratory virus on the incidence of respiratory disease in weaned beef calves. Prev Vet Med 2008;85:151–7.

Index

Note: Page numbers of article titles are in **boldface** type.

A

Adnexal pain, in farm animals, ocular squamous cell carcinoma and, 431–432
Age, as factor in OSCC, 518
Akinesia, in eye examination in ruminants and camelids, 438–439
Anesthesia/anesthetics
    in surgical treatment of eyes in farm animals, 473–474
    local, in eye examination in ruminants and camelids, 438–439
Anophthalmos, in production animals, 477–479
Anterior chamber, in eye examination in ruminants and camelids, 449–450

B

Blindness, in farm animals, congenital cataracts and, 432–433

C

Camelid(s)
    eye disorders in, therapeutic regimens for, 453–455
    eye examination in, **437–458.** See also *Eye examination, in ruminants and camelids.*
    South American, ophthalmology of, **531–555.** See also *South American camelids.*
Cataract(s), congenital
    in farm animals, blindness due to, 432–433
    in production animals, 481–483
Chemotherapy, in OSCC management, 523–525
Choroid, porcine, 561–565
Ciliary body, porcine, 561–565
Coloboma(s), optic nerve, in production animals, 483
Congenital abnormalities, in production animals, **477–486**
    anophthalmos, 477–479
    cataracts, 481–483
    cyclopia, 479–481
    gonotlo oauooo, 481
    infectious causes, 481
    microphthalmos, 477–479
    multiple disorders, 481
    optic nerve colobomas, 483
Congenital cataracts
    in farm animals, blindness due to, 432–433
    in production animals, 481–483
Conjunctiva
    disorders of, in South American camelids, 545–546
    in eye examination in ruminants and camelids, 446–447

Vet Clin Food Anim 26 (2010) 595–601
doi:10.1016/S0749-0720(10)00053-8
0749-0720/10/$ – see front matter © 2010 Elsevier Inc. All rights reserved.

vetfood.theclinics.com

Moving?

Make sure your subscription moves with you!

To notify us of your new address, find your **Clinics Account Number** (located on your mailing label above your name), and contact customer service at:

Email: journalscustomerservice-usa@elsevier.com

800-654-2452 (subscribers in the U.S. & Canada)
314-447-8871 (subscribers outside of the U.S. & Canada)

Fax number: 314-447-8029

Elsevier Health Sciences Division
Subscription Customer Service
3251 Riverport Lane
Maryland Heights, MO 63043

*To ensure uninterrupted delivery of your subscription, please notify us at least 4 weeks in advance of move.

Printed and bound by CPI Group (UK) Ltd, Croydon, CR0 4YY

03/10/2024

01040444-0013